Cancer Immunotherapy in Urology

Editors

SUJIT S. NAIR
ASHUTOSH K. TEWARI

UROLOGIC CLINICS
OF NORTH AMERICA

www.urologic.theclinics.com

Consulting Editor
SAMIR S. TANEJA

November 2020 • Volume 47 • Number 4

ELSEVIER

1600 John F. Kennedy Boulevard • Suite 1800 • Philadelphia, Pennsylvania, 19103-2899

http://www.theclinics.com

UROLOGIC CLINICS OF NORTH AMERICA Volume 47, Number 4
November 2020 ISSN 0094-0143, ISBN-13: 978-0-323-75498-9

Editor: Kerry Holland
Developmental Editor: Julia McKenzie

Urologic Clinics of North America (ISSN 0094-0143) is published quarterly by Elsevier Inc., 360 Park Avenue South, New York, NY 10010-1710. Months of issue are February, May, August, and November. Business and Editorial Offices: 1600 John F. Kennedy Blvd., Suite 1800, Philadelphia, PA 19103-2899. Periodicals postage paid at New York, NY and additional mailing offices. Subscription prices are $391.00 per year (US individuals), $795.00 per year (US institutions), $100.00 per year (US students and residents), $450.00 per year (Canadian individuals), $993.00 per year (Canadian institutions), $100.00 per year (Canadian students/residents), $520.00 per year (foreign individuals), $993.00 per year (foreign institutions), and $240.00 per year (foreign students/residents). Foreign air speed delivery is included in all *Clinics* subscription prices. All prices are subject to change without notice. **POSTMASTER:** Send address changes to *Urologic Clinics of North America*, Elsevier Health Sciences Division, Subscription Customer Service, 3251 Riverport Lane, Maryland Heights, MO 63043. **Customer Service: 1-800-654-2452 (US). From outside the United States, call 1-314-447-8871. Fax: 1-314-447-8029. E-mail: JournalsCustomerServiceusa@elsevier.com (for print support)** and **JournalsOnlineSupport-usa@elsevier.com (for online support)**.

Reprints. For copies of 100 or more, of articles in this publication, please contact the Commercial Reprints Department, Elsevier Inc., 360 Park Avenue South, New York, New York 10010-1710. Tel.: 212-633-3874; Fax: 212-633-3820; E-mail: reprints@elsevier.com.

Urologic Clinics of North America is covered in MEDLINE/PubMed (*Index Medicus*), *Excerpta Medica, Current Contents/Clinical Medicine, Science Citation Index,* and *ISI/BIOMED.*

Contributors

CONSULTING EDITOR

SAMIR S. TANEJA, MD
The James M. Neissa and Janet Riha Neissa
Professor of Urologic Oncology, Professor of
Urology, Radiology, and Biomedical
Engineering, GU Program Leader, Perlmutter
Cancer Center, Director, Division of Urologic
Oncology, Department of Urology, NYU
Langone Health, New York, New York, USA

EDITORS

SUJIT S. NAIR, PhD
Assistant Professor, Director of GU
Immunotherapy Research, Department of
Urology, Icahn School of Medicine at Mount
Sinai, New York, New York, USA

**ASHUTOSH K. TEWARI, MBBS, MCh, FRCS
(Hon)**
Professor and System Chair, The Milton and
Carroll Petrie Department of Urology, Director,
Center of Excellence for Prostate Cancer at the
Tisch Cancer Institute, Mount Sinai Health
System, Icahn School of Medicine at Mount
Sinai, New York, New York, USA

AUTHORS

JEANNY B. ARAGON-CHING, MD
GU Medical Oncology, Inova Schar Cancer
Institute, Fairfax, Virginia, USA

KRISTIN G. BEAUMONT, PhD
Assistant Professor, Genetics and Genomic
Sciences, Icahn School of Medicine at Mount
Sinai, Icahn Institute for Data Science and
Genomic Technology, New York, New York,
USA

MICHAEL A. BEAUMONT, PhD
Assistant Professor, Genetics and Genomics
Sciences, Icahn School of Medicine at Mount
Sinai, Icahn Institute for Data Science and
Genomic Technology, New York, New York,
USA

NINA BHARDWAJ, MD, PhD
Department of Hematology and Oncology,
Icahn School of Medicine at Mount Sinai, The

Tisch Cancer Institute, New York, New York,
USA

MARIJO BILUSIC, MD
Genitourinary Malignancies Branch, Center for
Cancer Research, National Cancer Institute,
Bethesda, Maryland, USA

JEFFREY M. BOCKMAN, PhD
Executive Vice President, Oncology Practice
Head, Cello Health Bio Consulting (Previously
Defined Health), Florham Park, New Jersey,
USA

DIMPLE CHAKRAVARTY, DVM, PhD
Department of Urology and the Tisch Cancer
Institute, Icahn School of Medicine at Mount
Sinai, New York, New York, USA

NIVEDITA CHOWDHURY, MS
Department of Oncology, Sidney Kimmel
Comprehensive Cancer Center, Department of

Pathology, Johns Hopkins University School of Medicine, Baltimore, Maryland, USA; Columbia Center for Translational Immunology, Columbia University Medical Center, New York, New York, USA

WILLIAM L. DAHUT, MD
Genitourinary Malignancies Branch, Center for Cancer Research, National Cancer Institute, Bethesda, Maryland, USA

CHARLES G. DRAKE, MD, PhD
Columbia Center for Translational Immunology, Department of Urology, Division of Hematology and Oncology, Herbert Irving Comprehensive Cancer Center, Columbia University Medical Center, New York, New York, USA

DAVID J. EINSTEIN, MD
Division of Medical Oncology, Beth Israel Deaconess Medical Center, Boston, Massachusetts, USA

ADAM M. FARKAS, PhD
Department of Hematology and Oncology, Icahn School of Medicine at Mount Sinai, The Tisch Cancer Institute, New York, New York, USA

ZEYNEP GUL, MD
Department of Urology, Icahn School of Medicine at Mount Sinai, New York, New York, USA

JAMES L. GULLEY, MD
Genitourinary Malignancies Branch, Center for Cancer Research, National Cancer Institute, Bethesda, Maryland, USA

LI HUANG, MD, PhD
Department of Urology, Icahn School of Medicine at Mount Sinai, New York, New York, USA; Department of Urology, Sun Yat-sen Memorial Hospital, Sun Yat-sen University, Guangzhou, China

KATHLEEN HWANG, MD
Department of Urology, University of Pittsburgh School of Medicine, Pittsburgh, Pennsylvania, USA

MATTHEW KAHN, MS
Department of Urology, Icahn School of Medicine at Mount Sinai, New York, New York, USA

FATIMA H. KARZAI, MD
Genitourinary Malignancies Branch, Center for Cancer Research, National Cancer Institute, Bethesda, Maryland, USA

KEVIN R. LOUGHLIN, MD, MBA
Harvard Medical School, Boston, Massachusetts, USA

RAVI A. MADAN, MD
Clinical Director, Genitourinary Malignancies Branch, Center for Cancer Research, National Cancer Institute, Bethesda, Maryland, USA

RANA McKAY, MD
Division of Hematology-Oncology, Department of Internal Medicine, University of California, San Diego, La Jolla, California, USA

J. KELLOGG PARSONS, MD, MHS
Department of Urology, University of California, San Diego, La Jolla, California, USA

DEVIN PATEL, MD
Department of Urology, University of California, San Diego, La Jolla, California, USA

ROBERT SEBRA, PhD
Associate Professor, Genetics and Genomic Sciences and Black Family Stem Cell Institute, Icahn School of Medicine at Mount Sinai, Icahn Institute for Data Science and Genomic Technology, New York, New York, USA' Sema4, a Mount Sinai venture, Stamford, Connecticut, USA

JOHN P. SFAKIANOS, MD
Department of Urology, Icahn School of Medicine at Mount Sinai, New York, New York, USA

SUSAN F. SLOVIN, MD, PhD
Attending Physician, Member, Genitourinary Oncology Service, Department of Medicine, Sidney Kimmel Center for Prostate and Urologic Cancers, Memorial Sloan Kettering Cancer Center, Professor of Medicine, Weill Cornell Medical College, New York, New York, USA

ASHUTOSH K. TEWARI, MBBS, MCh, FRCS (Hon)
Professor and System Chair, The Milton and Carroll Petrie Department of Urology, Director,

Center of Excellence for Prostate Cancer at the
Tisch Cancer Institute, Mount Sinai Health
System, Icahn School of Medicine at Mount
Sinai, New York, New York, USA

DANIELLE VELEZ, MD
Division of Urology, Department of Surgery,
Brown University, Providence, Rhode Island,
USA

Contents

William B. Coley: His Hypothesis, His Toxin, and the Birth of Immunotherapy   413

Kevin R. Loughlin

In recent years, immunotherapy has been the focus of great interest to researchers, clinicians, and the general public. Traditionally cancer therapy has been thought to be limited to surgery, radiation therapy, or chemotherapy. Some clinicians have considered it the so-called fifth pillar of cancer therapy, following surgery, cytotoxic chemotherapy, radiation, and targeted therapy. However, the origins of immunotherapy in cancer treatment reach back at least into the nineteenth century. This article reviews the origins, development, and future of immunotherapy.

Kidney Cancer: An Overview of Current Therapeutic Approaches   419

Nivedita Chowdhury and Charles G. Drake

The management of metastatic renal cell carcinoma (RCC) has evolved rapidly in recent years with several immunotherapy-based combinations of strategies approved as first-line therapies. Targeted strategies, including systemic antiangiogenesis agents and immune checkpoint blockade, form the basis of a therapeutic approach. With rising rates of recurrence after first-line treatment, it is increasingly important to not only adopt a personalized treatment plan with minimal adverse events but also develop predictive biomarkers for response. This review discusses currently available first-line and second-line therapies in RCC and their pivotal data, with specific focus on ongoing clinical trials in the adjuvant setting, including those involving novel agents.

Harnessing Natural Killer Cell Function for Genitourinary Cancers   433

Nina Bhardwaj, Adam M. Farkas, Zeynep Gul, and John P. Sfakianos

Natural killer (NK) cells are potently cytolytic innate lymphocytes involved in the immune surveillance of tumors and virally infected cells. Although much progress has been made in manipulating the ability of T cells to recognize and eliminate tumors, a comprehensive understanding of NK-cell infiltration into solid tumors, and their amenability to immunomodulation, remains incomplete. This article discusses recent studies showing that urologic tumors are infiltrated by NK cells and that these NK cells are often dysfunctional, but that strategies interfering with inhibitory axes have significant potential to alleviate this dysfunction.

Immunotherapy for Localized Prostate Cancer: The Next Frontier?   443

Devin Patel, Rana McKay, and J. Kellogg Parsons

Cancer vaccines, cytokines, and checkpoint inhibitors are immunotherapeutic agents that act within the cancer immunity cycle. Prostate cancer has provided unique opportunities for, and challenges to, immunotherapy drug development, including low tumor mutational burdens, limited expression of PD-L1, and minimal

T-cell intratumoral infiltrates. Nevertheless, efforts are ongoing to help prime prostate tumors by turning a "cold" prostate cancer "hot" and thus rendering them more susceptible to immunotherapy. Combination treatments, use of molecular biomarkers, and use of new immunotherapeutic agents provide opportunities to enhance the immune response to prostate tumors.

Biochemically recurrent prostate cancer represents a stage of prostate cancer where conventional (continued on next page) computed tomography and technetium Tc 99m bone scan imaging are unable to detect disease after curative intervention despite rising prostate-specific antigen. There is no clear standard of care and no systemic therapy has been shown to improve survival. Immunotherapy-based treatments potentially are attractive options relative to androgen deprivation therapy due to the generally more favorable side-effect profile. Biochemically recurrent prostate cancer patients have a low tumor burden and likely lymph node-based disease, which may make them more likely to respond to immunotherapy.

Multiple immunologic platforms have provided minimal impact in patients with metastatic castration-resistant prostate cancer, necessitating that novel approaches continue to be developed. Although checkpoint inhibitors have been largely ineffective, there remain small cohorts of patients who have durable responses but lack the conventional indicators for response to this class of drugs, that is, high mutational burden or significant genomic alterations, as seen in other solid tumors. This article presents an update on the evolution of immunotherapeutics that target a more lethal form of prostate cancer and provides the groundwork for future considerations as to how this field should proceed.

Cancer is a highly complex and heterogeneous disease and immunotherapy has shown promise as a therapeutic approach. The increased resolution afforded by single-cell analysis offers the hope of finding and characterizing previously underappreciated populations of cells that could prove useful in understanding cancer progression and treatment. Urologic and prostate cancers are inherently heterogeneous diseases, and the potential for single-cell analysis to help understand and develop immunotherapeutic approaches to treat these diseases is very exciting. In this review, we view cancer immunotherapy through a single-cell lens and discuss the state-of-the-art technologies that enable advances in this field.

The advent of immunotherapy has revolutionized cancer treatment. Prostate cancer has an immunosuppressive microenvironment and a low tumor mutation burden, resulting in low neoantigen expression. The consensus was that immunotherapy would be less effective in prostate cancer. However, recent studies have reported that prostate cancer does have a high number of DNA damage and repair gene defects. Immunotherapies that have been tested in prostate cancer so far have been mainly vaccines and checkpoint inhibitors. A combination of genomically targeted therapies, with approaches to alleviate immune response and thereby make the tumor microenvironment immunologically hot, is promising.

The age of immuno-oncology has ushered in a rush within the biopharmaceutical industry. This intense focus has been characterized as a frenzy or overhyped, but represents a substantial investment in new products that hope to harness the immune system against cancer. Such agents include next-generation checkpoint antagonists, immune costimulatory agonists, and a diverse array of novel mechanisms of action and therapeutic modalities targeting immune cell types and the interplay of the host and tumor at the immune synapse. This article surveys the clinical development and investment activity with Immuno-Oncology, specifically prostate, kidney, and bladder cancers.

Special Article

Personalized medicine uses a patient's genotype, environment, and lifestyle choices to create a tailored diagnosis and therapy plan, with the goal of minimizing side effects, avoiding lost time with ineffective treatments, and guiding preventative strategies. Although most precision medicine strategies are still within the laboratory phase of development, this article reviews the promising technologies with the greatest potential to improve the diagnosis and treatment options for male infertility, including sperm cell transplantation, genomic editing, and new biomarker assays, based on the latest proteomic and epigenomic studies.

UROLOGIC CLINICS OF NORTH AMERICA

SERIES OF RELATED INTEREST:
Hematology/Oncology Clinics of North America
http://www.hemonc.theclinics.com/

Preface

Immunotherapy for Genitourinary Cancers: New Opportunities for Clinical Impact

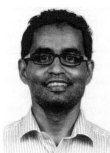
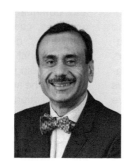

Sujit S. Nair, PhD   Ashutosh K. Tewari, MBBS, MCh, FRCS (Hon)

Editors

It would be an understatement to say that the concept of immunotherapy—the treatment of cancer through suppression or stimulation of the immune system—was slow to gain acceptance. A century passed between the publication of William B. Coley's report of a treatment for sarcoma employing "bacterial toxins" and the first Food and Drug Administration–approved immunotherapy in 1990, bacillus Calmette-Guérin (BCG) for bladder cancer. In the 30 years since, immunotherapy has revolutionized cancer treatment. Today, there are nearly 3 dozen approved immunotherapeutics for 20 different cancers, and despite ongoing challenges, advances in research have resulted in remarkable impact on clinical practice.

Immunotherapy in genitourinary (GU) cancers presents significant opportunities, especially in the context of recent breakthroughs. As the articles in this issue of *Urologic Clinics* describe, approvals of immune checkpoint blockade have changed the standard of care for advanced renal carcinomas, with a number of these strategies now approved as first- and second-line treatments. A growing body of evidence suggests that in biochemically recurrent prostate cancer, for which there is currently no current standard of care or systemic therapy, immune-based therapies may slow disease progression. Despite the persistent challenges prostate cancer creates for

immunotherapy drug development, pivotal clinical trials have pointed to potential combinations of therapies that may be effective, and new studies have highlighted the emerging role of immunotherapy for localized prostate cancer. Novel combinations of immunotherapies have also shown promise in both early- and late-stage bladder cancers, particularly in patients who have not responded well to BCG.

The articles in this issue highlight breakthroughs, as well, in our understanding of the biology of urologic tumors. Recent studies have shown that natural killer (NK) cells infiltrate urologic tumors and that these cells are often dysfunctional. Preclinical data and research in human cells have demonstrated the potential of immunotherapeutic interventions to alleviate this dysfunction, and diverse NK-cell-centric clinical trials are underway in bladder, kidney, and prostate cancers. In addition, in prostate cancer specifically, other next-gen immunotherapy approaches that exploit the prostate-specific lineage surface protein targets are a compelling and growing new area: bispecific T-cell engagers, antibody-drug conjugate therapy, and third-generation chimeric antigen receptor T cells.

Development of targeted cell and gene therapies will benefit greatly from the advent of single-cell sequencing, which will help address one of the most challenging aspects of understanding

Urol Clin N Am 47 (2020) xi–xii
https://doi.org/10.1016/j.ucl.2020.08.001
0094-0143/20/© 2020 Published by Elsevier Inc.

and treating cancer—heterogeneity. Single-cell sequencing technologies make it possible to characterize the key contributions to the disease of specific cell subpopulations in both the tumor and the tumor microenvironment (TME), including a network of noncancerous cells types and extracellular matrix proteins outside of the tumor that may contribute to disease progression. The complexity of the TME has only recently been appreciated but will be extremely important moving forward, especially in delineating the distinctions between urologic cancers. Given their immunologically distinct TME, better understanding of the TME in bladder and prostate cancers will be critical for successful development of intratumoral neoadjuvant immunotherapy approaches that target early cancer clones before they have modified the tumor environment.

Identification of subpopulations of cells in the TME will enable identification of new therapeutic targets and disease biomarkers and ultimately enable better understanding of why some patients respond to a particular therapy while others do not. Understanding differentiated response to treatment has, arguably, been one of the most complex and perplexing aspects of immunotherapy. While such immunotherapies as checkpoint blockade have resulted in a paradigm shift in disease management, the fact remains, nonetheless, that cancer is not cured in the majority of patients, and both academic and industry investigators are sharply focused on discovery and testing of novel combinations of therapies.

As described in this issue, immuontherapy in metastatic settings remains especially challenging. Genomic approaches will enable better understanding of "lethal" phenotypes, specifically in the case of prostate cancer, and of metastatic disease across GU cancers, and will support discovery of novel biomarkers for the development of targeted approaches. Preclinical animal models may be especially useful for advancing such strategies. Finally, much work continues to develop a more nuanced understanding of the intricacies of the innate immune system in the context of GU cancers, specifically, the mechanisms that play a role in the activation of immunity or in immune escape.

These review articles demonstrate the need for, and potential of, targeted and customized approaches, cancer by cancer, and patient by patient. They demonstrate the promise of novel combinatorial strategies in the context of better understanding of the complex biology of GU cancers and the advent of innovative tools for analysis and prediction. We hope this special issue, with 13 articles, including 4 online-only articles, has conveyed the realistic and not insubstantial challenges and significant opportunities for GU cancer immunotherapy.

Sujit S. Nair, PhD
Department of Urology
Icahn School of Medicine at Mount Sinai
Annenberg 24-15
New York, NY 10029, USA

Ashutosh K. Tewari, MBBS, MCh, FRCS (Hon)
Department of Urology
Icahn School of Medicine at Mount Sinai
Mount Sinai Health System
One Gustave L. Levy Place
Box 1272 L6-57
New York, NY 10029, USA

E-mail addresses:
Sujit.nair@mountsinai.org (S.S. Nair)
Ash.tewari@mountsinai.org (A.K. Tewari)

William B. Coley
His Hypothesis, His Toxin, and the Birth of Immunotherapy

Kevin R. Loughlin, MD, MBA

KEYWORDS

- William B. Coley • Toxin • Immunotherapy • Cancer

KEY POINTS

- At the end of the 19th century, William B. Coley introduced the concept of immunotherapy.
- He observed dramatic responses of tumor regression in some patients following would infection.
- His theories were largely discredited and ignored for over a century.

INTRODUCTION

In recent years, immunotherapy has been the focus of great interest to researchers, clinicians, and the general public. Traditionally cancer therapy has been thought to be limited to cut, burn, and poison, or surgery, radiation therapy, or chemotherapy.[1] Some clinicians have considered it the so-called fifth pillar of cancer therapy, following surgery, cytotoxic chemotherapy, radiation, and targeted therapy.[2] However, the origins of immunotherapy in cancer treatment reach back at least into the nineteenth century. This article reviews the origins, development, and future of immunotherapy.

EARLY IMMUNOTHERAPY

In the mid-1800s 2 German physicians, Busch and Fehleisen,[3] independently observed regression of tumors in patients with cancer after accidental infections by erysipelas.[2] In 1868, Busch[29] intentionally infected a patient with cancer with erysipelas and noted shrinkage of the tumor. In 1882, Fehleisen[3] repeated this treatment and identified *Streptococcus pyogenes* as the causative agent of erysipelas.

WILLIAM B. COLEY: "THE MOST OPPORTUNE TIME IN A THOUSAND YEARS"

William B. Coley was a young surgeon in New York City in 1890 who had recently graduated from Harvard Medical School. Coley[1] thought that he had entered medicine at the "most opportune time in a thousand years." He was about to meet a young female patient who would change his career and would affect the future of cancer treatment.

Elizabeth "Bessie" Dashiell was a 17-year-old friend of John D. Rockefeller Jr. In the summer of 1890, she returned from a cross-country train trip with what appeared to be a minor injury of her right hand, which she had caught in the seat lever of her Pullman rail car. Because of her ongoing pain, Rockefeller suggested that she see Doctor Coley. On examination, he noted some swelling and discoloration. He incised the mass and found no obvious infection and sent her home with a diagnosis of periostitis.

She returned when her condition did not improve, and Coley operated a second time and performed a biopsy. The biopsy returned as a sarcoma. She had a rapid downhill course with metastases to her breast, liver, and abdomen, and soon died.

Bessie's rapid demise was not only upsetting to Coley but spurred him to investigate whether this was an unusual clinical course for a sarcoma. Coley began to review the records of all the previous patient with sarcoma at New York Hospital. One record caught his attention. Seven years earlier, a 31-year-old patient named Fred Stein had been seen at New York Hospital with a large

Harvard Medical School, Boston, MA, USA
E-mail address: kloughlin@partners.org

Urol Clin N Am 47 (2020) 413–417
https://doi.org/10.1016/j.ucl.2020.07.001

left neck mass that had been proved to be a sarcoma. One of the attending surgeons had operated on the mass, but it recurred. Stein underwent 5 operations over the course of 3 years. He required skin grafts, which failed, and he ultimately developed a wound infection with erysipelas (S pyogenes). Erysipelas was frequently the cause of virulent postoperative infections in that period and had been referred to as St Anthony's fire since the Middle Ages.[1]

Stein had never returned for follow-up and Coley was curious what had happened to him. After some medical sleuthing, Coley was ultimately able to track down Stein living on the Lower East Side of Manhattan. On examination and having Stein further evaluated at New York Hospital, it appeared that Stein was free of disease 7 years after his original diagnosis. Why had these 2 patients with sarcoma had such different outcomes? Coley wondered whether the wound infection had played a role.

In 1891, Coley saw another patient, known only as Mr Zola, with a recurrent sarcoma of the neck. It was deemed inoperable. Based on his previous experience, Coley thought that injecting Zola's tumor with erysipelas was worth a try, given the circumstances. The tumor appeared to slough, but did not totally disappear. Coley was encouraged.

Coley surmised that he needed to induce a more severe infection and that the extent of the febrile response might be a good marker. Through contacts, he was able to obtain what was thought to be a more potent bacterial brew from Robert Koch in Berlin. With further injections of the new preparation, Mr Zola's tumor totally regressed without recurrence after 8.5 years of follow-up.

These early experiences led Coley to hypothesize that the infection elaborated a substance or substances that caused the tumors to regress. One of Coley's challenges was that the preparation of his "toxin" was arbitrary without a standard formula or concentration. Coley's toxin was ultimately a mixture of S pyogenes and Serratia marcescens. Coley 's results were inconsistent: some patients responded and some did not.

At the same time, he was experiencing some political problems. The head of the New York Cancer Hospital (which would ultimately become Memorial Sloan Kettering Cancer Center), James Ewing, was skeptical of Coley's work and was also very enthusiastic about the new modality of radiation therapy. Coley's work remained controversial.

From 1923 to 1963, Parke-Davis was the only source of Coley's toxins in the United States. In 1963, the Food and Drug Administration (FDA) assigned Coley's toxin to a new-drug status, which made it illegal to prescribe it outside of clinical trials. The mechanism of action of the toxins was never fully elucidated. Because the activity of the toxins was associated with fever, it was thought that it resulted from a lipopolysaccharide that increased lymphocyte activity and boosted tumor necrosis factor (TNF).[4] However, Tsung and Norton[5] have reported that the active agent is interleukin-12, rather than TNF.

BACILLI CALMETTE-GUÉRIN: UROLOGY'S IMMUNOTHERAPY SUCCESS STORY

In the early part of the twentieth century, tuberculosis (TB) continued to be a major public health issue. TB is caused by Mycobacterium tuberculosis and Mycobacterium bovis, which are known collectively as tubercle bacilli.[6] In 1908, Albert Calmette, a bacteriologist, and Camille Guérin, a veterinarian, working together at the Pasteur Institute, began trying to develop a TB vaccine. They isolated a virulent strain of M bovis from an infected cow and, after passages though multiple cultures, showed gradual loss of virulence. In 1921, after 231 passages in subcultures through 13 years, they showed attenuation to a nonvirulent, but genetically stable, form in guinea pigs.[6]

This unique strain of M bovis was named after Calmette and Guérin and became known as bacilli Calmette-Guérin (BCG). They first tested the BCG on a baby whose mother and grandmother had TB. The baby had no side effects and did not develop TB. From 1921 to 1924, 217 Parisian children were vaccinated with BCG and were successfully immunized against TB.[6]

It had been noted that TB seemed to have antitumor effects. In 1929, Pearl,[7] through an autopsy study at Johns Hopkins Hospital, reported a lower frequency of cancer in patients with TB. He went on to show that cancer survivors had a higher incidence of active or healed TB than individuals dying of cancer. He concluded that there was some type of protection against cancer conferred by TB, but could not explain a mechanism.

In 1930, because of a laboratory error, a large number of German babies were vaccinated with contaminated BCG and died. This incident was known as the Lubeck Disaster and decreased the enthusiasm for BCG as a cancer therapy for the next 3 decades.[6]

In 1959, the next major advance in the understanding of the mechanism of action of BCG occurred. Old and colleagues[8] reported that mice infected with BCG showed increased resistance to a challenge with transplantable tumors. BCG caused general augmentation of immunologic activity and was found to activate macrophages that inhibited or destroyed cancer cells. This finding was the first direct evidence of the antitumor effects of BCG, which became known as TNF.

In the 1970s, Zbar and colleagues[9] defined the criteria for successful BCG therapy, which included (1) close contact between BCG and the tumor cells, (2) a host capable of mounting an immunologic response to mycobacterial antigens, (3) a limited burden, and (4) adequate numbers of viable BCG organisms.

In 1972, Morales and colleagues[10] initiated the original BCG protocol for bladder cancer treatment, which was 6 weekly treatments of 120 mg in 50 mL of saline instilled via a urethral catheter. An intradermal injection of BCG was performed to assess delayed hypersensitivity injection. The initial trail of 10 patients showed no bladder cancer recurrences in the 47 patient months of follow-up after BCG treatment.[10]

In 1975, de Kernion and colleagues[11] reported that an isolated melanoma in the bladder was successfully treated with cystoscopic injection of BCG vaccine. In 1978, Morales received approval from the National Cancer Institute to fund 2 randomized trials to test the effectiveness of the combined BCG regimen against superficial bladder cancer.[12,13] More data continued to accrue to support the efficacy of BCG in the treatment of superficial bladder cancer. In 1990, the FDA approved the general use of intravesical BCG for the treatment of noninvasive bladder cancer.

THE LANDMARKS OF IMMUNOLOGIC DISCOVERY THAT PROVIDED THE FOUNDATION FOR IMMUNOTHERAPY

Over the past decades, there have been robust, fundamental scientific discoveries that have laid the foundation for the new era of immunotherapy treatment of malignancy. A summary of some of the major landmarks is provided in **Table 1**.

Interferon was discovered in 1957 by Issacs and Linderman.[14] Interferons are naturally occurring substances that interfere with the ability of viruses to reproduce, and they also boost the immune system. There are 3 classes of interferons: alpha, beta, and gamma. In therapeutic doses, interferons may have significant side effects. Although they only have a minor role in modern immunotherapy, their discovery provided insight into some of the natural immune responses of the body.

Besides interferon, other cytokines have generated clinical interest. Interleukin-2 (IL-2) and interferon-alpha have shown mild clinical benefits

Table 1 Landmarks of immunotherapy and cancer treatment	
1868	Wilhelm Busch reports impact of erysipelas on a tumor
1891	William B. Coley begins his investigations using his toxin
1957	Discovery of interferon by Alick Isaacs and John Lindenmann
1959	Immune surveillance cancer theory by Lewis Thomas and F.M. Burnet
1959	Chemical structure of antibodies by Gerald Edelmann and Sidney Porter
1974	Cell-mediated immunity described by Peter Doherty and Rolf Zinkermagel
1975	Monoclonal antibodies manufactured by Caser Milstein and George Koehler
1975	Discovery of TNF by Lloyd Old
1982	Discovery of T-cell receptor by James Allison, B. McIntyre, and D. Bloch
2011	First anti–CTLA-4 drug (ipilimumab). First checkpoint inhibitor approved by FDA
2012	Discovery of CRISPR/Cas9 system: more efficient method of genome editing
2018	Nobel Prize awarded to James Allison and Tasuko Honjo for discovery of cancer therapy by inhibition of negative immune regulation

Abbreviations: CRISPR, clustered regularly interspaced short palindromic repeat; CTLA, cytotoxic T lymphocyte–associated protein.

and have received FDA approval for the treatment of several cancers. IL-2 was approved for the treatment of advanced renal cell carcinoma and metastatic melanoma, and interferon-alpha was approved for hairy cell leukemia, follicular non-Hodgkin lymphoma, melanoma, and acquired immunodeficiency syndrome–related Kaposi sarcoma. The application of these cytokines was a milestone in cancer immunotherapy because it showed that immunotherapy could achieve durable, objective clinical responses.

Immune surveillance was a concept that was proposed by Burnet and Thomas[15–17] in the late 1950s. Every day, each cell in the body is estimated to experience more than 20,000 DNA-damaging events,[2,18] which are normally repaired without sequelae.[2,19] Cells that are not repaired and that acquire malignant potential are then usually recognized and killed by the tumor immunosurveillance system.[2] This concept that the immune system is capable of identifying and killing nascent nonself malignant cells was a major milestone in thinking and was developed by Burnet[15,17] and Thomas.[16] It provided the underpinning for the construct of immunoediting processes, which are divided into elimination, equilibrium, and escape.[2] Hanahan and Weinberg[20] proposed 8 hallmarks of cancer, and the ability of cancer cells to evade immune destruction has been identified as the eighth hallmark of cancer.

Adoptive cell therapy is another form of immunotherapy that involves the isolation and in vitro expansion of tumor-specific T cells.[2] The FDA has approved anti–cluster of differentiation (CD) 19 chimeric antigen receptor (CAR) T cells[21,22] as well as cultures of tumor-infiltrating T lymphocytes.[23] These approaches apply strategies that depend on cytokines for in vitro expansion and in vivo persistence of transferred T cells.

Berraondo and colleagues[21] propose that the search for the next generation of cytokine-based drugs is based on 3 concepts. First, synergistic combinations of anti–programmed cell death protein 1 (PD-1) and programmed death-ligand 1 (PD-L1) monoclonal antibodies and CAR 19 T cells. Second, improved pharmacokinetics, whereby the half-lives of cytokines could be increased in the circulation. Third, achieving higher local concentrations of cytokines into the tumor microenvironment with recombinant proteins[24] or gene therapy vectors.[25,26]

CHECKPOINT INHIBITORS

The most recent advance in cancer immunotherapy has been the discovery and clinical applications of immune checkpoint inhibitors, anti–cytotoxic T lymphocyte–associated protein 4 (CTLA-4), PD-1, and PD-L1, which provide a strategy to modulate the immune system to fight the malignancy. These drugs remove the "brakes" on the immune system and permit T-cell activation.[27,28]

Studies have been published and more are ongoing using a variety of immune checkpoint inhibitors in prostate cancer, renal cancer, and bladder cancer. Ipilimumab, the first monoclonal directed against CTLA-4, has been used to treat prostate cancer. T cells require 2 signals to become fully activated. CD28 and CTLA-4 are T-cell receptors that play a decisive role in initial activation and subsequent control of cellular immunity.[29] Ipilimumab has been used in several prostate cancer trials and 2 studies deserve mention. One study, CA184-095, randomized (2:1) 602 men who were chemotherapy naive to ipilimumab or placebo. Although progression-free survival was longer in the ipilimumab arm, the results showed that the therapy had no effect on overall survival.[30] A second study, CA184-043, compared ipilimumab with placebo in 799 men with metastatic castration-resistant prostate cancer previously treated with radiotherapy and docetaxel chemotherapy. There was no improvement in overall survival (hazard ratio [HR], 0.85; $P = .53$), but there was a suggestion of benefit in patients with more favorable disease.[31]

In November 2015, nivolumab (anti–PD-1) received FDA approval for the treatment of patients with metastatic renal cell carcinoma who had progressed on antiangiogenic therapy. In a phase 3 study, CheckMate 025, 821 patients with advanced renal cell carcinoma who had 1 or 2 prior tyrosine kinase inhibitors were randomized to treatment with nivolumab or everolimus. Although progression-free survival was similar between the groups, the primary end point of overall survival favored nivolumab rather than everolimus (25 months vs 19.6 months; HR, 0.73, $P = .002$). Interestingly, the survival benefit did not depend on the expression of PD-L1 on tumor cells.[32]

The most extensive experience with checkpoint inhibitor drugs in urologic oncology has been in the treatment of bladder cancer. A variety of anti–PD-1 and anti–PD-L1 agents, atezolizumab (IMvigor210), durvalumab (phase 1/2 study 1108), pembrolizumab (KEYNOTE-045), nivolumab (CheckMate-275), and avelumab (JAVELIN) have all been FDA approved for the treatment of urothelial carcinoma in patients pretreated or relapsed with platinum-based therapy since 2016 or 2017. Multiple ongoing phase 3 investigations are in progress.

The underpinnings of the scientific discoveries that have laid the foundation for the exciting era of cancer immunotherapy date back for more than a century. It is not hyperbole to state that the next decade offers the potential for clinical advances in cancer care that have never been imagined. Malignancies once thought to be incurable will realistically be curable. The potential for progress in immunotherapy is limitless.

REFERENCES

1. Graeber C. The breakthrough: immunotherapy and the race to cure cancer. New York: Twelve Publishing; 2018. p. 1, 37, 41.
2. Oiseth SJ, Aziz MS. Cancer immunotherapy: a brief review of the history, possibilities and challenges ahead. J Cancer Metastasis Treat 2017;3:250–61.

3. Fehleisen F. Velerdie Zuch der Erysipelkokken auf kunstlichem Nohrboden und ihre Ubertrogbarkert auf den Menschen. Dtsch Med Wochenschr 1882; 88:553–4.

4. Coley's Toxins. Wikipedia. Available at: http://en.wikipedia.org/wiki/Coley'sToxins. Accessed October 31, 2019.

5. Tsung K, Norton A. Lessons from Coley's Toxin. Surg Oncol 2006;15(1):25–8.

6. Herr HW, Morales A. History of bacillus calmette-guerin and bladder cancer: an immunotherapy success story. J Urol 2008;179:53–6.

7. Pearl R. Cancer and tuberculosis. Am J Hyg 1929;9: 97.

8. Old LJ, Clark DA, Benacerrof B. Effect of bacillus Calmette-Guerin infection on transplanted tumors in the mouse. Nature 1959;184:291.

9. Zbar B, Bernstein ID, Rapp HJ. Suppression of tumor growth at the site of infection with living bacillus Calmette-Guerin. J Natl Cancer Inst 1971;46:831.

10. Morales A, Eidinger D, Bruce AW. Intracavitary bacillus Calmette-Guerin in the treatment of superficial bladder tumors. J Urol 1976;116:180.

11. De Kernion JB, Golub SH, Gupta RK, et al. Successful transurethral intralesional BCG therapy of a bladder melanoma. Cancer 1975;36:1662.

12. Lamm DL, Thor DE, Harris SC, et al. Bacillus Calmette-Guerin. Immunotherapy of Superficial Bladder Cancer. J Urol 1980;124:38.

13. Camacho FJ, Pinsky CM, Herr HW, et al. Treatment of superficial bladder cancer with intravesical BCG. Proc Am Soc Clin Oncol 1980;21:359.

14. Issacs A, Lindenmann J. Virus interference. The interferon. Proc R Soc Lond B Biol Sci 1957;147: 258–67.

15. Burnet M. Cancer: a biological approach III. Viruses associated with neoplastic conditions IV. Br Med J 1957;1:841–7.

16. Thomas L. Discussion. In: Lawrence HS, editor. Cellular and humoral aspects of the hypersensitive state. New York: Hoeber-Harper; 1959. p. 524–32.

17. Burnet FM. The concept of immunological surveillance. Prog. Exp. Tumor Res 1970;13:1–27.

18. Loeb LA. Human cancers express mutator phenotypes: origin, consequences and targeting. Nat Rev Cancer 2011;11:450–7.

19. Lindahl T, Wood TD. Quality control by DNA repair. Science 1999;286:1897–905.

20. Hanahan D, Weinberg RA. Hallmarks of cancer: the next generation. Cell 2011;144:646–74.

21. Berraondo P, Sanmamed MF, Ochoa MC, et al. Cytokines in clinical cancer immunotherapy. Br J Cancer 2018;120:6–15.

22. June CH, O'Connor RS, Kawalekar OU, et al. CAR T cell immunotherapy for human cancer. Science 2018;359:1361–5.

23. Hinriohs CS, Rosenberg SA. Exploiting the curative potential of adoptive T cell therapy for cancer. Immunol Rev 2014;257:56–71.

24. Jackaman C, Bundell CS, Kinnear BF, et al. IL-2 intratumoral immunotherapy enhances CD8+T cells that mediate destruction of tumor cells and tumor-associated vasculature: a novel mechanism for IL-2. J Immunol 2003;171: 5051–63.

25. Sangro B, Mazzolini G, Ruiz J, et al. Phase 1 trial of intratumoral injection of an adenovirus encoding interleukin-12 for advanced digestive tumors. J Clin Oncol 2004;22:1389–97.

26. Hu J, Sun C, Bernatchez C, et al. T cell homing therapy for reducing regulatory T cells and preserving T cell function in large solid tumors. Clin Cancer Res 2018;24:2920–34.

27. Meng, MV, Boughey JC. Bulletin of the American College of Surgeons 8/2/17.

28. Janiczek M, Szylberg L, Kasperska A, et al. Immunotherapy as a promising treatment for prostate cancer: a systematic review. J Immunol Res 2017. https://doi.org/10.1155/2017/4861570. Accessed April 22, 2019.

29. Busch W. Aus der Sitzung der mediaischen Section vom 13 November 1867. Berlin: Klin Wochenschor; 1868. p. 5137 [in German].

30. Beer TM, Kwan ED, Drake CG, et al. Randomized, double-blind, phase III trial of ipilimumab versus placebo in asymptomatic or minimally symptomatic patients with metastatic, chemotherapy-naïve, castration-resistant prostate cancer. J Clin Oncol 2017;35:40.

31. Kwan ED, Drake CG, Scher HI, et al. Ipilimumab versus placebo after radiotherapy in patients with metastatic, castration-resistant prostate cancer that had progressed after docetaxel chemotherapy (CA 184-043): A multicenter , randomized, double blinded, phase 3 trial. Lancet Oncol 2014;15(7): 7001.

32. Obara W, Kato R, Kato Y, et al. Recent progress in immunotherapy for urologic cancer. Int J Urol 2017;24(10):735.

Kidney Cancer
An Overview of Current Therapeutic Approaches

Nivedita Chowdhury, MS[a,b,c], Charles G. Drake, MD, PhD[c,d,e],*

KEYWORDS

- Kidney cancer • Clear cell carcinoma • First-line immunotherapy • Tyrosine kinase inhibitors
- Atezolizumab • Pembrolizumab • Bevacizumab

KEY POINTS

- Recent approvals of immune checkpoint blockade have changed the standard of care for advanced renal carcinomas, ushering a new era of combination therapy.
- Improved first-line and second-line treatments are being investigated to reduce the risk of recurrence among patients with advanced disease.
- Upcoming treatment strategies involve new tyrosine kinase inhibitors, novel combinations, and alternative agents to improve targeted therapy.

INTRODUCTION

Worldwide, approximately 400,000 individuals were diagnosed with renal cell carcinoma (RCC) in 2018; that is, it is fairly common. In the United States, RCC is among the top 10 most common cancers, with a notable increase in incidence over the past several years.[1] For localized (organ-confined) disease, surgical resection potentially is curative. Unfortunately, 25% to 30% of patients present with distant metastatic disease at the time of diagnosis[2]; and approximately 40% of surgically resected patients eventually develop recurrence.[3]

The 2 pillars of therapy for metastatic RCC (mRCC), vascular endothelial growth factor (VEGF) tyrosine kinase inhibitors (TKIs) that attenuate progression by inhibiting angiogenesis,[4] and immunotherapy, predominantly in the form of agents that block the immune checkpoint mediated by the interaction between Programmed cell death protein 1 (PD-1) on tumor-specific T cells and programmed death ligand 1 (PD-L1) expressed on either tumor cells or myeloid cells in the tumor microenvironment (TME) (**Fig. 1**). TKIs are broadly effective, with several agents, including sorafenib,[5] sunitinib,[6] pazopanib,[7] and cabozantinib,[8] approved in the first-line setting. More recent studies established combination regimes as the preferred front-line treatment, that is, the combination of anti–PD-1 (nivolumab) plus Cytotoxic T-lymphocyte associated protein

Conflict of Interest: C.G. Drake is a coinventor on patents licensed from Johns Hopkins to BMS and Janssen; has served as a paid consultant to AZ Medimmune, BMS, Compugen, Pfizer, Roche, Sanofi Aventis, Genentech, Merck, and Janssen; and has received sponsored research funding to his institution from the Bristol-Myers Squibb International Immuno-Oncology Network. N. Chowdhury declares no conflicts.

a Department of Oncology, Sidney Kimmel Comprehensive Cancer Center, Johns Hopkins University School of Medicine, Baltimore, MD 21287, USA; b Department of Pathology, Johns Hopkins University School of Medicine, Baltimore, MD 21287, USA; c Columbia Center for Translational Immunology, Columbia University Medical Center, 177 Fort Washington Avenue, Suite 6GN-435, New York, NY 10032, USA; d Department of Urology, Herbert Irving Comprehensive Cancer Center, Columbia University Medical Center, 177 Fort Washington Avenue, Suite 6GN-435, New York, NY 10032, USA; e Division of Hematology and Oncology, Herbert Irving Comprehensive Cancer Center, Columbia University Medical Center, 177 Fort Washington Avenue, Suite 6GN-435, New York, NY 10032, USA
* Corresponding author. 177 Fort Washington Avenue, Suite 6GN-435, New York, NY 10032.
E-mail address: cgd2139@cumc.columbia.edu

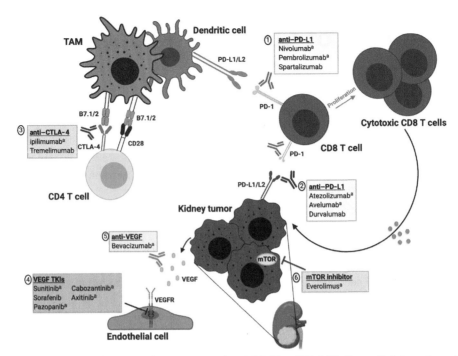

Fig. 1. Current molecular and immunotherapy targets in mRCC. ICIs of PD-1 (1) disrupt its interaction with PD-L1, leading to enhanced T-cell proliferation and activation. Antibodies targeting PD-L1 (2) prevent its interaction with PD1 on CD8 T cells, allowing their activation. Anti–CTLA-4 (3) antibodies allow CD28 to bind to its receptor, B7.1/2, and activate naïve CD4 T cells. Antiangiogenesis targets include TKIs (4) on VEGFR and the anti-VEGF monoclonal antibody, bevacizumab (5). Lastly, mTOR inhibitors (6) prevent tumor growth. TAM, tumor-associated macrophage. [a] FDA approved.

4 (CTLA)-4 (ipilimumab) for intermediate-risk and high-risk patients,[9] and the combination of anti–PD-1 (pembrolizumab) or anti–PD-L1 (avelumab) plus axitinib for patients regardless of performance status.[10,11] When anti–PD-1 or anti-PD-L1 is used in the first-line setting, second-line monotherapy[12] with anti–PD-1 is illogical, so current second-line regimens include monotherapy with agents that were not used in the first line (cabozantanib or axitinib) or the combination of the TKI lenvatinib with the mammalian target of rapamycin (mTOR) inhibitor everolimus.[13–15]

Given the relatively high rate of recurrence after surgery for primary, organ-confined disease, post-surgical (adjuvant) TKI therapy was tested in several phase III trials; these generally have been less than overwhelmingly successful.[16] More recent trials are testing the role of anti–PD-1 or anti–PD-L1 in the adjuvant setting; but those are long-term studies for which data are not yet available. Based on strong preclinical data[17] and some clinical data[18] showing an enhanced clinical benefit for immunotherapy prior to surgery (neoadjuvant immunotherapy), there are several ongoing neoadjuvant immunotherapy trials in RCC, including smaller trials aimed at understanding

the biological effects of a given treatment or combination as well as a pivotal trial[19] (NCT03055013), testing whether the combination of neoadjuvant plus adjuvant immunotherapy improves progression-free survival (PFS) in surgically resected patients. Taken together, these data highlight the rapidly evolving clinical status of RC, as well as the interesting biological questions currently being addressed.

FIRST-LINE COMBINATION THERAPIES FOR METASTATIC RENAL CELL CARCINOMA
Combined Immune Checkpoint Blockade

As discussed previously, immune checkpoint blockade (ICB) involves blocking the interaction between immune checkpoint molecules on T cells and their ligands, which are expressed on either tumor cells or myeloid cells in the TME.[20] ICB thus reverses the exhausted phenotype of cytotoxic T cells, enhancing their ability to mount a tumor-specific immune response. Nivolumab and pembrolizumab are anti–PD-1 antibodies preventing its interaction with PD-L1/2, whereas the monoclonal antibodies atezolizumab, avelumab, and durvalumab block PD-L1. The other major immune checkpoint involved in immunosuppression in the RCC TME is CTLA-4, which when expressed binds avidly to B7-1 and B7-2, thus inhibiting signal 2 and preventing full T-cell activation.[21] Based on the activity of PD-1 blockade in the second-line setting[12] as well as on preclinical data[22] and melanoma,[23] a phase III study (Checkmate 214)[9] was completed in treatment-naïve mRCC. This study compared combination immunotherapy with ipilimumab and nivolumab to standard-of-care treatment with the TKI sunitinib. The trial enrolled patients with all risk categories, but, based on previous data suggesting improved activity in patients with intermediate-risk and poor-risk disease, the primary endpoints were focused on intermediate-risk and poor-risk patients. The study met its primary endpoint, showing that intermediate-risk/poor-risk patients had an improved median PFS of 11.6 months versus 8.4 months (hazard ratio [HR] 0.82; $P = .03$), respectively, and an objective response rate (ORR) of 42% versus 27%, respectively, compared with sunitinib alone, regardless of PD-L1 expression. Patients with PD-L1 expression greater than 1% showed better PFS (HR 0.46; 95% CI, 0.31-0.67) and complete response (CR), 16% vs 7%, respectively, than patients with less than 1% PD-L1 expression. Perhaps most significantly, 9% of the patients treated with combination immunotherapy experienced a CR as opposed to 1% in the sunitinib arm. After 25.2 months of follow-up, the median OS was not yet reached for the combination and was 18.2 months in patients treated with sunitinib alone. Discontinuation of the study due to toxicity was higher (22% vs 8%, respectively) for combination immunotherapy than for sunitinib alone,[12] but patients on combination immunotherapy surprisingly reported a better quality of life compared with sunitinib. For patients with favorable-risk disease, sunitinib showed an improved PFS (HR 2.18; 99.1% CI, 1.29-3.68; $P<.001$) and ORR (52% vs 29%, respectively) compared with the combination therapy. As a result, the combination therapy was approved as a first-line treatment of intermediate-risk/poor-risk advanced RCC, supporting the rationale for combination immunotherapy in mRCC. Although these data (especially the rate of CRs) are impressive, the activity of this combination regimen needs to be balanced with its significant rate of immune-related adverse events (AEs) (approximately 60%).

Combining Immune Checkpoint Blockade with Tyrosine Kinase Inhibitors

RCC is a highly vascular disease with hallmark overexpression of hypoxia- inducible factor (HIF) 1a (as a result of von Hippel-Lindau tumor suppressor gene inactivation) and its downstream targets, predominantly VEGF. Several small molecule inhibitors of VEGF are currently Food and Drug Administration (FDA)-approved for RCC; these include sorafenib,[5] sunitinib,[6] pazopanib,[7] and axitinib,[24] among others.[25] These agents inhibit tumor angiogenesis, thus resulting in objective tumor responses in some cases and in disease stabilization in others. As a class, VEGF blocking agents generally are associated with several adverse events, including fatigue, hand-foot syndrome, bleeding, and rash.[25] A majority of recent trials in the first-line setting use sunitinib as a comparator arm; this is reasonable because its pivotal trial showed improved overall survival (OS) (26.4 months vs 21.8 months, respectively; HR 0.821; 95% CI, 0.673–1.001) and ORR of 47% compared with 12% for IFNγ, alone.[6]

Sunitinib and sorafenib are perhaps dirty TKIs, in that they inhibit multiple TKs beyond VEGF. More recently, axitinib, a more selective inhibitor of VEGF receptor (VEGFR)-1, VEGFR-2, and VEGFR-3, was tested for its antiangiogenesis activity in a phase III trial for treatment-naïve mRCC patients. Initial data suggested no significant increase in median PFS compared with sorafenib.[26] Subsequent follow-up, however, revealed a similar safety profile and OS (21.7 months vs 23.3 months, respectively) as sorafenib,[27] on the whole, with a better OS (41.2 months vs 31.9 months, respectively) in patients with a good Eastern Cooperative Oncology Group (ECOG) performance status.

Because of their clear activity in RCC, combining VEGF TKI with anti–PD-1 seemed to be a logical next step in combination therapy. Initial efforts in this regard were not particularly successful; one arm of a trial combining anti–PD-1 (nivolumab) with the TKI pazopanib was halted due to excessive liver toxicity.[28] A similar result was observed when pazopanib was combined with pembrolizumab, even when the agents were administered sequentially.[29] The combination of sunitinib plus nivolumab was slightly better tolerated, but further development of that combination was not pursued, perhaps in favor of the anti–CTLA-4 plus anti–PD-1 combination, discussed previously.

The TKI axitinib appears to be a far better tolerated combination partner for immunotherapy, possibly because of its greater selectivity for VEGFR downstream signaling. A single-armed phase Ib trial combining axitinib with pembrolizumab[10] showed the combination to be generally well tolerated, with an ORR of 73% (95% CI, 59.0–84.4). The rate of grade III/IV AEs was significant, at approximately 60%, although a majority of these involved hypertension, an expected AE for axitinib.[24] Based on these results, a phase III trial (Keynote-426[10]) was initiated in treatment-naïve mRCC patients. Here, the combination showed a longer median PFS (15.1 months vs 11.1 months, respectively; HR 0.69; 95% CI, 0.57–0.84; P<.001), ORR (59.3% vs 35.7%, respectively); and 12-month OS rate of 83.4% versus 79.5%, respectively, compared with sunitinib alone. This was consistent in patients from favorable-risk, intermediate-risk, and poor-risk groups and irrespective of PD-L1 expression. These data led to the approval of the combination of pembrolizumab/axitinib as a first-line treatment in previously untreated mRCC patients.

Axitinib also has been tested in combination with the anti–PD-L1 antibody avelumab in PD-L1 positive, treatment-naïve patients, leading to the recent approval of the first anti–PD-L1 therapy against mRCC in a combination setting.[11] The phase III trial (JAVELIN Renal 101) showed a median PFS of 13.8 months versus 7.2 months, respectively (HR 0.61; 95% CI, 0.47–0.79; P<.001), compared with sunitinib alone, in patients with PD-L1–positive tumors (63.2%). The combination ORR was significantly higher, at 55.2% versus 25.5%, respectively, with a median OS of 11.6 months versus 10.7 months, respectively, for sunitinib. The rate of adverse events was comparable in both arms of the study, with grade 3 or higher in 71.2% and 71.5% of the patients, respectively.

Taken together, these 3 trials established combination immunotherapy as a default treatment strategy for first-line RCC. The ipilimumab/nivolumab combination is appropriate for patients with intermediate-risk and high-risk disease, whereas the axitinib plus avelumab is appropriate for patients with PD-L1–positive tumors. The axitinib plus pembrolizumab combination is broadly approved and can be used regardless of risk group or PD-L1 status. Although combination immunotherapy produces impressive response rates and provides a clear improvement in PFS (and likely OS) compared with TKI monotherapy, all 3 of these combination regimens are associated with a significant rate of grade III/IV AE, and none has a rate of CRs greater than 20%, highlighting a need for further improvement.

Combination Therapy with Anti–Vascular Endothelial Growth Factor Antibodies

Bevacizumab is a monoclonal antibody that targets VEGF-A; it has shown a significant effect on survival and response in solid tumors, including RCC.[30] A phase III trial (IMmotion151) compared combination treatment with atezolizumab plus bevacizumab versus sunitinib alone in patients with PD-L1 expression.[31] The median PFS was 11.2 months versus 7.7 months, respectively (HR 0.74; 95% CI, 0.57-0.96; P<.0217), in combination compared with sunitinib alone. The improved PFS was maintained in all subtypes of PD-L1 expressing tumors, including liver metastases and favorable-risk groups. The median OS had an HR of 0.93 in the intention-to-treat population, with a favorable safety profile (8% vs 5%, respectively; discontinued treatment due to adverse events). Longer follow-up currently is under way for more definitive OS data, but bevacizumab + atezolizumab currently is not FDA approved for RCC. Thus, as with moving toward improving the outcomes and survival data for patients with metastatic disease (**Table 1**), these new immunotherapy combinations most likely are the standard-of-care treatment of most metastatic RCC patients.

SECOND-LINE TREATMENT STRATEGIES FOR METASTATIC RENAL CELL CARCINOMA

Because few mRCC patients obtain a CR to first-line treatment, even with the potent immunotherapy combinations, discussed previously, a majority of patients with mRCC progress and are treated with second-line therapy. Although anti–PD-1 (nivolumab) previously was favored in the second line, the evolving treatment landscape, in which an anti–PD-1 or anti-PD-L1 agent is used in the first-line means that second-line treatment with immunotherapy monotherapy no longer is clinically advisable, that is, based on mechanism of action, it is highly unlikely that patient who progresses on axitinib + pembrolizumab, axitinib + avelumab, or ipilimumab + nivolumab will respond to nivolumab monotherapy. Thus, currently favored second-line regimens include cabozantinib and axitinib monotherapy. Some first-line RCC patients with slowly progressing RCC still are treated initially with TKI monotherapy; for such patients, nivolumab monotherapy remains an appropriate second-line regimen (**Table 2**).

Cabozantinib

Cabozantinib, a TKI targeting multiple tyrosine kinases, including VEGFR, MET, and AXL, has been tested in treatment-naïve mRCC patients as well as in a second-line treatment setting. The up-regulation of MET and AXL as a result of VHL inactivation has been linked with poor outcome.[34] Cabozantinib initially was approved for use in mRCC patients who had progressed on prior treatment with another TKI. A phase III trial (METEOR)

Table 1
Study data and survival outcomes from key studies for first-line treatment of renal cell carcinoma

	Combination Therapies				Monotherapy	
	Nivolumab + Ipilimumab	Pembrolizumab + Axitinib	Avelumab + Axitinib	Atezolizumab + Bevacizumab	Sunitinib	Cabozantinib
Trial	CheckMate 214[9]	Keynote-426[10]	Javelin 101[11]	IMmotion151[31]	SUTENT[6]	CABOSUN[8]
N	861	886	1096	915	750	157
Median follow-up (mo)	25.2	12.8	12	24	11	34.5
ORR	39.0%[a]	59.3%[a]	51.4%[a]	37.0%[a]	47%	33%
CR	10.2%[a]	5.8%[a]	3.4%[a]	5.0%[a]	3%	NA
PFS (mo) Combination arm	12.4	15.1	13.8	11.2	Treatment arm 11	8.6
Sunitinib arm	12.3	11.1	8.4	8.4	IFN-α or sunitinib arm 5	5.3
HR (CI)	**0.85** (95% CI, 0.73–0.98)	**0.69** (95% CI, 0.57–0.84)	**0.69** (95% CI, 0.56–0.84)	**0.83** (9% CI, 0.70–0.97)	**0.539** (95% CI, 0.45–0.64)	**0.48** (95% CI, 0.31–0.74)
OS (mo) Combination arm	NR	NR	NR	33.6	Treatment arm 26.4	26.6
Sunitinib arm	37.9	NR	NR	34.9	IFN-α or sunitinib arm 21.8	21.2
HR (CI)	**0.71** (95% CI, 0.59–0.86)	**0.53** (95% CI, 0.38–0.74)	0.78 (95% CI, 0.55–1.08)	0.93 (95% CI, 0.76–1.14)	**0.821** (95% CI, 0.67–1.01)	0.8 (95% CI, 0.53–1.21)

HR with statistically significant CIs are in bold.
Abbreviation: NR, not reached.
a ORR and CR rate in combination immunotherapy arm.

Table 2
Study data and survival outcomes from currently approved second-line treatments for metastatic renal cell carcinoma

		Nivolumab	Cabozantinib	Axitinib
Trial		CheckMate 025[12]	METEOR[32]	AXIS[33]
N		821	658	698
Median follow-up (mo)		25.2	18.7	26.5
ORR		25%	17%	52% (in favorable-risk)
CR		1%	NA	—
PFS (mo)	Treatment arm	4.6	13.8	8.3
	Other arm	Everolimus, 4.4	Everolimus, 8.4	Sorafenib, 5.7
	HR (CI)	0.88	**0.51**	**0.656**
		(95% CI, 0.75–1.03)	(95% CI, 0.41–0.62)	(95% CI, 0.55–0.78)
OS (m)	Treatment arm	25	21.4	20.1
	Other arm	Everolimus, 19.6	16.5	19.2
	HR (CI)	**0.73**	**0.66**	0.969
		(98.5% CI, 0.57–0.93)	(95% CI, 0,53–0,83)	(95% CI, 0,8–1,17)

HR with statistically significant CIs are in bold.
Data from Refs.[12,32,33]

compared cabozantinib to everolimus in TKI-refractory mRCC tumors. Improved median PFS (HR 0.51; 95% CI, 0.41–0.62), OS (HR 0.66; 95% CI, 0.53–0.83), and ORR (17% vs 3%, respectively) were seen in patients treated with cabozantinib compared with everolimus.[32] Importantly, patients with bone metastases showed significant responses to cabozantinib. Based on these data, a phase II trial (CABOSUN) was initiated, comparing it to sunitinib in the first-line setting for mRCC patients with intermediate-risk/poor-risk disease. Cabozantanib significantly improved PFS (HR 0.66; 95% CI, 0.46–0.95; P<.012) along with an ORR of 20% versus 9%, respectively, compared with sunitib.[8] The PFS benefit was seen in all patients, regardless of presence of bone metastases. Tumors with MET expression responded better to cabozantinib compared with MET tumors, indicating a potential additive effect of targeting both VEGFR and MET simultaneously. In the second-line setting (after first-line combination treatment), a phase II trial BREAKPOINT (NCT03463681) of cabozantinib after prior treatment with ICB currently is ongoing, with a preliminary reported increase in PFS from 3.8 months to 7.4 months.[14] Based on these results, cabozantinib likely will continue to be used in second-line.

Cabozantanib also is being tested, however, in the first-line setting as a combination partner with nivolumab. Results from a phase I study (NCT02496208) of using cabozantinib in combination with nivolumab with or without ipilimumab were presented at American Society of Clinical Oncology:Genitourinary Cancer Symposium 2018.[35] These data showed ORR of 54% in the RCC patients within a cohort of genitourinary tumors. Long-term response and benefit remain to be seen. A phase III study (CheckMate 9ER) tested the combination of cabozantinib/nivolumab in patients with treatment-naïve mRCC versus sunitinib alone.[36] The study recently completed has enrollment although details have not yet been published. If the cabozantanib/nivolumab regimen is used in the first line, then second-line treatment likely would involve axitinib or the lenvantinib/everolimus combination.

Axitinib

As discussed previously, the VEGF-specific TKI axitinib was evaluated in a phase III trial (AXIS) comparing second-line axitinib versus the TKI sorafenib. This trial enrolled mRCC patients with favorable risk/intermediate risk and no bone or liver metastases.[33] The AXIS trial was the first phase III study to compare 2 VEGF-based therapies in mRCC. The PFS was improved in patients treated with axitinib for both favorable-risk and intermediate-risk patients. The median PFS was 13.9 months versus 4.7 months, respectively (HR 0.476; 95% CI, 0.263–0.863; P = .0126), and less than 5 months versus less than 2 months, respectively (HR 0.378; 95% CI, 0.195–0.734; P = .0032), in favorable-risk versus poor-risk mRCC patients. No benefit in OS was seen in either treatment arm (20.1 months vs 19.2 months, respectively). Based on the longer PFS and safety profile, axitinib was approved as a second-line treatment in mRCC. Axitinib performed better in patients with favorable risk and, thus, is a suitable treatment option for them. For patients who are treated with avelumab/axitinib or pembrolizumab/axitinib in the first line, axitinib is not a sensible second-line treatment option. Axitinib remains a viable treatment option, however, for patients treated with either ipilimumab/nivolumab, or with a monotherapy with a different TKI. More recent data from a phase II trial (NCT02579811) of 40 patients treated with individualized axitinib after prior treatment with ICB, revealed a median PFS as 8.8 months with an ORR of 45%,[13] supporting its activity in the second-line setting.

Immune Checkpoint Blockade: Nivolumab Monotherapy

ICB has shown better outcomes and survival data compared with other therapies in solid tumors, such as melanoma.[23] An open-label, phase III trial (CheckMate 025) in bevacizumab refractory mRCC patients compared nivolumab to everolimus (mTOR inhibitor, considered standard first-line treatment in patients, where targeting VEGF failed and with good survival data). There was an improvement in the median OS of 25 months versus 19.6 months, respectively (HR –0.72, $P<.02$) and ORR of 21.5% versus 3.9%, respectively, in patients treated with nivolumab. This was the first trial showing better survival data in a second-line setting for mRCC.[12] Not only did more patients respond to nivolumab, but also the duration of response was higher (23 months vs 13.7 months, respectively) than in those treated with everolimus. With 19% of the patients showing grade 3/4 adverse events (Compared with 37% in patients treated with everolimus), nivolumab was considered to have a modest safety profile and was approved by the FDA as a second-line treatment of mRCC patients. As discussed previously, at the current time, most mRCC patients likely receive an anti–PD-1 or anti–PD-L1 agent in the first-line setting; for such patients, second-line treatment with nivolumab monotherapy is not appropriate.

ADJUVANT TREATMENT IN RENAL CELL CARCINOMA

For RCC patients with localized tumors, frontline treatment involves the removal of the tumor via surgical resection and subsequent active surveillance. As discussed previously, 20% to 40% of patients recur after surgery.[3] The relatively high rate of recurrence suggests that many localized RCC patients have micrometastatic disease at the time of surgery and that treating these micrometastases with an appropriate agent might lead to an improved PFS and perhaps OS. One challenge with adjuvant studies in RCC is that there currently are no reliable prognostic biomarkers for recurrence in RCC. Some factors, such as VHL mutation status, PD-L1 expression, and presence of bone metastases, may affect the treatment strategy and use of TKIs, anti–PD-L1 immune checkpoint inhibitors (ICIs), and cabozantinib, respectively. These data, however, are based on single-armed studies and have not been broadly validated. Based on the relatively high rate of recurrence after primary therapies, several of the TKIs were tested in the adjuvant setting; several of these trials have been completed and published.[16,25]

Adjuvant Therapy with Tyrosine Kinase Inhibitors

Treatment with the TKIs, sorafenib, pazopanib, and sunitinib, in the adjuvant setting has been studied in SORCE, PROTECT, and S-TRAC, respectively. SORCE was a randomized placebo-controlled study testing sorafenib in patients with high-risk to intermediate-risk RCC after resection. After 3 years of treatment, no difference in PFS or OS was seen.[37] Additionally, no differences in 5-year and 10-year disease-free survival (DFS) rates were noted (67% vs 65%, respectively, and 54% vs 53%, respectively) and it was concluded that sorafenib is not appropriate as an adjuvant therapy for RCC. A similar result was observed in PROTECT, a phase III trial of adjuvant pazopanib in patients with localized RCC having a high risk of recurrence. After 12 months, DFS was slightly favorable for pazopanib (HR 0.86; 95% CI, 0.70–1.06) but pazopanib treatment did not show any significant improvement.[38] S-TRAC was a multi-institutional, placebo-controlled phase III study testing sunitinib for a year after surgery in patients with high risk of recurrence. Unlike SORCE and PROTECT, median DFS for S-TRAC was 6.8 years versus 5.6 years, respectively (HR – 0.76; 95% CI, 0.59–0.98; 2-sided P = .03).[39] Grade 3/4 AES were more common in the sunitinib arm compared with the placebo group (48.4% for grade 3 and 12.% for grade 4 vs 15.8% and 3.6%, respectively). Even though the toxicity was higher in the sunitinib arm, no deaths were recorded. These data led to the approval of sunitinib as an adjuvant treatment in RCC, although current practice patterns suggest that the agent rarely is used in this setting.

Immune Checkpoint Blockade in the Adjuvant Setting

RCC is an immunogenic tumor, and enhanced understanding of T-cell function and associated inhibitory molecules has led to the use of monoclonal antibodies, including anti–CTLA-4 (ipilimumab[9]), anti-PD1 (pembrolizumab[10] and nivolumab[9,12,40]), and anti-PD-L1 (atezolizumab[31] and avelumab[11]). Disease progression usually occurs to distant sites via circulating tumor cells and micrometastases from residual disease. As such, efficient adjuvant therapy is based on the notion that initiating an immune response targeting micrometastases may be optimized when the tumor burden is lowest, that is, after surgery. One unique benefit of adjuvant trials is that collection of primary tumors offers the opportunity to potentially determine biomarkers associated with recurrence (in the placebo arms) as well as predictive biomarkers for response (in the treatment arms).

The phase III trial, IMmotion010 (NCT03024996), evaluates the efficacy of atezolizumab (anti-PD-L1) in the adjuvant treatment of RCC based on its success as first-line therapy in bladder cancer[41] as well as in RCC (phase III IMmotion151[31] study, discussed previously) with an ORR of 43%. IMmotion010 enrolls PD-L1–positive patients with intermediate-risk to high-risk disease postnephrectomy. The study is limited to clear cell RCC with or without sarcomatoid dedifferentiation. The primary endpoint of this trial is DFS; as is the case for most adjuvant trials, it likely will be some time before results are reported.[42] Additional adjuvant trials evaluating other ICIs include pembrolizumab (anti-PD1, KEYNOTE-564 [NCT03142334][43]); and the combination of ipilimumab (anti-CTLA4) with nivolumab (anti-PD1) the adjuvant setting (CheckMate 914 [NCT03138512][44]). Both these trials currently are ongoing with a primary endpoint of DFS.

Lastly, the PROSPER study is an ECOG randomized, multi-institutional phase III study (NCT03055013) testing neoadjuvant and adjuvant therapy with nivolumab in patients with either node-positive tumors or stage T2–T4 compared with observation.[19] With recurrence-free survival as the primary readout, this study is based on the notion that nivolumab will more efficiently prime the immune system with the primary tumor in place, consistent with key data in preclinical models showing vastly enhanced activity for neoadjuvant immunotherapy compared with adjuvant immunotherapy.[17] This study also will provide an opportunity to determine the presence of PD-L1 expression is a predictive biomarker in clear cell as well as non–clear cell RCC. Adjuvant nivolumab will ensure continued exposure to ICI compared with surgery alone. This study currently is ongoing and plans to enroll approximately 800 participants to determine the effect of neoadjuvant nivolumab on clinical outcome and OS. The reason for the innovative design is 2-fold. First, the mechanism ICI suggests that a more robust antitumor immune response is elicited in the presence of the primary tumor. Thus, administration of presurgical nivolumab theoretically should amplify its efficacy in the adjuvant setting. Second, it enables the collection of tumor tissue before and after administration of nivolumab in this treatment-naïve cohort. This will further facilitate molecular characterization of RCC that may differentiate between patients who do and do not respond to therapy. Tertiary objectives of the PROSPER trial will be to correlate PD-L1 on both the primary tumor, and tumor tissue at recurrence, with clinical outcomes.

NEOADJUVANT THERAPY IN RENAL CELL CARCINOMA

Neoadjuvant therapy differs from adjuvant therapy in 1 ways: (1) timing, that is, prior to surgical resection (preoperative therapy); and (2) target—because surgery removes primary tumor, there is no indication on whether the residual cells or micrometastases include immune subsets, such as T cells, that can be modulated by ICB or, alternatively, express immune checkpoints. Moreover, advanced RCC patients with no feasible primary surgical approach may be amenable to a neoadjuvant approach. Previously, neoadjuvant strategies, including chemotherapy, targeted therapy, and ICB, have been successful in melanoma,[45] providing the basis to adapt a similar strategy against RCC. A recent study on 2 preclinical models of metastatic breast cancer elucidated the improved efficacy of neoadjuvant anti-PD1 by eradicating metastases and increasing tumor-specific CD8 T-cell response in peripheral blood.[17] These data provide a strong rationale to extensively test the neoadjuvant approach in RCC. There currently are 3 phase I clinical trials from different groups, which are evaluating the effect of nivolumab and pembrolizumab in a neoadjuvant setting: NCT02595918 (nivolumab, mRCC, and non-mRCC patients), NCT02575222 (nivolumab, tumor stages T2–T4), and NCT02212730 (pembrolizumab, RCC). In addition, the authors' group currently is working on 2 neoadjuvant studies in patients with treatment-naïve localized or locally advanced RCC (**Table 3**).

SPARC-1

In addition to their potential therapeutic benefit, neoadjuvant studies provide an ideal platform to interrogate the precise biological effects a given treatment exerts in the RCC TME. As an example, preclinical studies showed that proinflammatory cytokines, such as interleukin (IL)-1ß, may induce

Table 3
Currently ongoing clinical trials for neoadjuvant and adjuvant therapies in treatment of metastatic renal cell carcinoma

Treatment	Phase	National Clinical Trial Identification identifier	Estimated Completion Date
Perioperative nivolumab with adjuvant nivolumab (PROSPER)	III	NCT03055013	November 2023
Nivolumab as a neoadjuvant before surgery	I	NCT02595918	April 2021
Nivolumab as a neoadjuvant before surgery in high-risk patients	I	NCT02575222	June 2020 (no results yet)
Pembrolizumab as a neoadjuvant before surgery	I	NCT02212730	July 2019 (no results yet)
Spartalizumab in combination with anti–IL-1ß (canakinumab) prior to surgery in patients with localized RCC (SPARC-1)	I	NCT04028245	December 2021
Nivolumab/cabozantinib combination before undergoing cytoreductive surgery in mRCC (Cyto-KIK)	I	NCT04322955	February 2027

myeloid-derived suppressor cells (MDSCs), leading to immune suppression in the TME.[46] The authors' group has used a mouse tumor model for RCC to determine the effects of targeting IL-1ß (David H. Aggen, MD, PhD, unpublished data, 2020). Treatment with canakinumab (anti–IL-1ß) depleted the perimorphonuclear MDSCs within the tumor myeloid compartment ($0.76\% \pm -0.21$ vs vehicular control: $1.89\% \pm -0.37$; $P = .014$), without affecting the T-cell frequency.[47] Moreover, combining canakinumab with anti–PD-1 led to

reduction in tumor burden. With the success of anti–PD-1 ICIs and combination therapy in patients with advanced RCC, the authors initiated an early phase I study to incorporate spartalizumab in combination with anti–IL-1ß (canakinumab) prior to surgery in patients with localized RCC (NCT04028245) (**Fig. 2**). Spartalizumab targets PD-1 and prevents its interaction with PD-L1/L2, leading to activation of tumor-specific T-cell–mediated response. Spartalizumab currently is being tested in a phase I trial for colorectal cancer

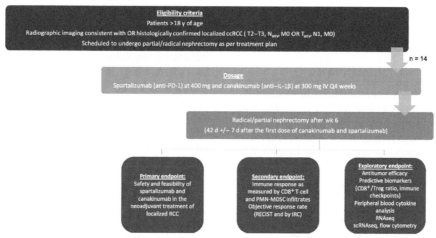

Fig. 2. Study design for SPARC-1 trial. ccRCC, clear cell renal carcinoma; IRC, immune-related response criteria; IV, intravenously; RECIST, response evaluation criteria in solid tumors; RNAseq, RNA sequencing; TNM Staging, tumor stage, node involvement, metastasis; Treg, regulatory T cells; PMN-MDSC, polymorphonuclear myeloid derived suppressor cells; scRNAseq, single-cell RNA sequencing.

(NCT04294160) and a phase III trial for melanoma (NCT02967692). Thus, the authors hypothesize that combination of PD-1 blockade with canakinumab can decrease the immunosuppressive MDSCs, inducing antitumor immune response in patients with localized RCC.

Combining Immunotherapy with Cytoreductive Nephrectomy—the CytoKIK Study

Although cytoreductive surgery alone has successfully improved survival[48] whereas TKI + surgery has not provided significantly better results,[49] the preliminary findings of the nivolumab/cabozantinib combination therapy suggest that priming the immune system might enhance the response further. As such, the authors' group hypothesized that use of this combination in a neoadjuvant setting would increase the number of patients with visible kidney cancer lesions during treatment. To test this hypothesis, the authors recently initiated a phase II trial, Cyto-KIK (NCT04322955) in treatment-naïve mRCC patients, where they will be treated with nivolumab/cabozantinib combination before undergoing cytoreductive surgery. The authors also intend to profile the immune microenvironment at the time of surgical resection to predict biomarkers of resistance to immunotherapy.

FUTURE DIRECTIONS

Combination therapies have proved feasible and are imminent to being approved as frontline as well as second-line treatment in mRCC. Additionally, determining the sequence of given treatment is of utmost importance and is dependent on various factors, including tumor stage, risk stratification, patient age, metastatic site, and Fuhrman grade, among others.

Sequential Order of Treatment

Although ICB-based combinations are standard of care for most patients with mRCC, currently, there is no optimal sequence of treatment of mRCC patients. As such, several groups are studying the effects of changing the order of the treatment on patient survival. A phase III study (COSMIC-313) of cabozantinib in combination with nivolumab and ipilimumab (triplet) followed by nivolumab/ipilimumab or matched placebo is ongoing. This trial includes previously untreated mRCC patients with intermediate-risk/poor-risk disease. The objective is to test the triplet combination and evaluate the PFS, with OS and ORR as secondary endpoints (NCT03937219). Another phase III study

(PDIGREE [NCT03793166]) compares the combination of nivolumab/ipilimumab followed by either nivolumab alone or a combination of nivolumab/cabozantinib in intermediate-risk/poor-risk patients with advanced RCC. Evaluating OS as the primary endpoint of the trial, it is believed that the combination of cabozantinib/nivolumab will improve the OS compared with nivolumab alone. Median PFS and ORR will be measured as secondary endpoints.

Emerging Immunotherapy Targets in Metastatic Renal Cell Carcinoma

Several evolving immunotherapy agents currently are in phase I and phase II trials; these recently have been reviewed.[50] Agents of interest include the following.

NKTR-214 (Pegylated Interleukin-2)

A recent study demonstrated that high-dose IL-2 results in a complete response in 1%, an objective response in 25%, and a partial response in 22% of patients with RCC.[51] Effector T cells generally express the IL-2 β/γ receptor[37], which, when targeted, may enhance the proliferative effect of IL-2 on T cells. NKTR-214, a polyethene glycol complexed prodrug binds to CD122, a subunit of IL-2R, stimulating an increased immune response. In an ongoing phase I/II trial of NTRK-214 plus nivolumab, responses were noted in 46% (6 of 13) of patients, with a disease control rate of 85% (11 of 13 patients).[52] These results from a small number of patients highlights the clinical potential of NKTR-214 in RCC therapy.

Adenosine A2A Receptor Drugs

Binding of adenosine, a purine nucleotide to its receptor, adenosine A2A receptor (A2AR), can have variable immunosuppressive effects by increasing regulatory T cells, inducing differentiation of M2 macrophages, and inhibiting natural killer cell function.[53] A small molecule ciforadenant (CPI-444, Corvus Pharmaceuticals, Burlingame, CA), targeting A2AR on T lymphocytes, currently is under study in a phase I trial [NCT02655822] evaluating the safety and tolerability of ciforadenant alone as well as in combination with atezolizumab in solid tumors, including RCC.

Glutaminase Inhibitor

Metabolic changes, especially in glucose and glutamine levels, lead to tumor development and survival in many cancers, including RCC. As such, a glutaminase inhibitor, telaglenastat, which inhibits proliferation in preclinical models of RCC, is being tested in combination with everolimus (phase II ENTRATA [NCT03163667]), cabozantinib (phase II, CANTATA [NCT03428217]), and nivolumab (phase I/II [NCT02771626]). With a tolerable safety profile, OS has not been reached for any of the trials but preliminary data for ENTRATA show an improved median PFS of 3.8 months versus 1.9 months, respectively, in telaglenastat/everolimus compared with matched placebo with everolimus.[54]

HIF2a Inhibitors

As a highly vascular disease, RCC usually develops with the overexpression of the oncogenic driver, HIF2a and its downstream targets, including VEGF. Targeting of HIF2a thus provides a promising therapeutic strategy to prevent the development of RCC. PT2977, an HIF2a inhibitor, is being tested alone (NCT03401788) as well as in combination with cabozantinib (NCT03634540) in patients with advanced RCC.[55] Of the 55 patients involved, 13 (24%) showed partial response whereas 31 (56%) had stable disease. The median PFS was 11 months (95% CI, 6–17), and the 12-month PFS rate was 49%.[56] The safety profile of PT2977 currently is unknown and is being investigated in these phase II trials.

SUMMARY

With the approval of multiple combination therapies for patients with mRCC, the standard-of-care practices, including first-line and second-line treatments, have transformed recently. There is, of course, a need for prognostic markers of recurrence and/or progression for better understanding of the TME. Absence of a consensus on order of treatment further complicates the standardization of the most optimal treatment strategy for each patient. With the results from some of the ongoing clinical trials involving more combination therapies, it is expected to shed some light on to the most effective and tolerable immunotherapy-based treatment.

FUNDIND SOURCES

Columbia University Irving Medical center, and Prostate Cancer Foundation.

REFERENCES

1. Bray F, Ferlay J, Soerjomataram I, et al. Global cancer statistics 2018: GLOBOCAN estimates of incidence and mortality worldwide for 36 cancers in 185 countries. CA Cancer J Clin 2018;68(6): 394–424.
2. Gupta K, Miller JD, Li JZ, et al. Epidemiologic and socioeconomic burden of metastatic renal cell carcinoma (mRCC): a literature review. Cancer Treat Rev 2008;34(3):193–205.
3. Kim SH, Park B, Hwang EC, et al. Retrospective multicenter long-term follow-up analysis of prognostic risk factors for recurrence-free, metastasis-free, cancer-specific, and overall survival after curative nephrectomy in non-metastatic renal cell carcinoma. Front Oncol 2019;9:859.
4. Rini BI. Vascular endothelial growth factor–targeted therapy in renal cell carcinoma: current status and future directions. Clin Cancer Res 2007;13(4): 1098–106.
5. Escudier B, Eisen T, Stadler WM, et al. Sorafenib in advanced clear-cell renal-cell carcinoma. N Engl J Med 2007;356(2):125–34.
6. Motzer RJ, Hutson TE, Tomczak P, et al. Overall survival and updated results for sunitinib compared with interferon alfa in patients with metastatic renal cell carcinoma. J Clin Oncol 2009; 27(22):3584.
7. Sternberg CN, Davis ID, Mardiak J, et al. Pazopanib in locally advanced or metastatic renal cell carcinoma: results of a randomized phase III trial. J Clin Oncol 2010;28(6):1061–8.
8. Choueiri TK, Hessel C, Halabi S, et al. Cabozantinib versus sunitinib as initial therapy for metastatic renal cell carcinoma of intermediate or poor risk (Alliance A031203 CABOSUN randomised trial): Progression-free survival by independent review and overall survival update. Eur J Cancer 2018; 94:115–25.
9. Motzer RJ, Tannir NM, McDermott DF, et al. Nivolumab plus ipilimumab versus sunitinib in advanced renal-cell carcinoma. N Engl J Med 2018;378(14): 1277–90.
10. Rini BI, Plimack ER, Stus V, et al. Pembrolizumab plus axitinib versus sunitinib for advanced renal-cell carcinoma. N Engl J Med 2019;380(12): 1116–27.
11. Motzer RJ, Penkov K, Haanen J, et al. Avelumab plus axitinib versus sunitinib for advanced renal-cell carcinoma. N Engl J Med 2019;380(12): 1103–15.
12. Motzer RJ, Escudier B, McDermott DF, et al. Nivolumab versus everolimus in advanced renal-cell carcinoma. N Engl J Med 2015;373(19):1803–13.
13. Ornstein MC, Pal SK, Wood LS, et al. Individualised axitinib regimen for patients with metastatic renal cell carcinoma after treatment with checkpoint inhibitors: a multicentre, single-arm, phase 2 study. Lancet Oncol 2019;20(10):1386–94.
14. Verzoni E, Bearz A, Giorgi UD, et al. A phase II open-label study of cabozantinib in patients with

advanced or unresectable renal cell carcinoma pretreated with one immune-checkpoint inhibitor: The BREAKPOINT trial. J Clin Oncol 2019;37(7_suppl): TPS685.

15. Motzer RJ, Hutson TE, Glen H, et al. Lenvatinib, everolimus, and the combination in patients with metastatic renal cell carcinoma: a randomised, phase 2, open-label, multicentre trial. Lancet Oncol 2015;16(15):1473–82.

16. Pal SK, Haas NB. Adjuvant therapy for renal cell carcinoma: past, present, and future. Oncologist 2014; 19(8):851–9.

17. Liu J, Blake SJ, Yong MCR, et al. Improved efficacy of neoadjuvant compared to adjuvant immunotherapy to eradicate metastatic disease. Cancer Discov 2016;6(12):1382–99.

18. Amaria RN, Menzies AM, Burton EM, et al. Neoadjuvant systemic therapy in melanoma: recommendations of the International Neoadjuvant Melanoma Consortium. Lancet Oncol 2019;20(7):e378–89.

19. Harshman LC, Puligandla M, Haas NB, et al. PROSPER: A phase III randomized study comparing perioperative nivolumab (nivo) versus observation in patients with localized renal cell carcinoma (RCC) undergoing nephrectomy (ECOG-ACRIN 8143). J Clin Oncol 2019;37(7_suppl):TPS684.

20. Drake CG, Lipson EJ, Brahmer JR. Breathing new life into immunotherapy: review of melanoma, lung and kidney cancer. Nat Rev Clin Oncol 2013;11:24.

21. Sharma P, Allison James P. Immune checkpoint targeting in cancer therapy: toward combination strategies with curative potential. Cell 2015;161(2): 205–14.

22. Korman A, Chen B, Wang C, et al. Activity of Anti-PD-1 in Murine Tumor Models: Role of "Host" PD-L1 and synergistic effect of anti-PD-1 and Anti-CTLA-4 (48.37). J Immunol 2007;178(1 Supplement):S82.

23. Wolchok JD, Chiarion-Sileni V, Gonzalez R, et al. Overall survival with combined nivolumab and ipilimumab in advanced melanoma. N Engl J Med 2017;377(14):1345–56.

24. Hutson TE, Gallardo J, Lesovoy V, et al. Axitinib versus sorafenib as first-line therapy in patients with metastatic renal cell carcinoma (mRCC). Journal of clinical Oncology 2013;31(6).

25. Gul A, Rini BI. Adjuvant therapy in renal cell carcinoma. Cancer 2019;125(17):2935–44.

26. Hutson TE, Lesovoy V, Al-Shukri S, et al. Axitinib versus sorafenib as first-line therapy in patients with metastatic renal-cell carcinoma: a randomised open-label phase 3 trial. Lancet Oncol 2013; 14(13):1287–94.

27. Hutson TE, Al-Shukri S, Stus VP, et al. Axitinib versus sorafenib in first-line metastatic renal cell carcinoma: overall survival from a randomized phase III trial. Clin Genitourin Cancer 2017;15(1):72–6.

28. Goodman AM, Kato S, Bazhenova L, et al. Tumor mutational burden as an independent predictor of response to immunotherapy in diverse cancers. Mol Cancer Ther 2017;16(11):2598–608.

29. Chowdhury S, McDermott DF, Voss MH, et al. A phase I/II study to assess the safety and efficacy of pazopanib (PAZ) and pembrolizumab (PEM) in patients (pts) with advanced renal cell carcinoma (aRCC). J Clin Oncol 2017;35(15_suppl):4506.

30. Roviello G, Bachelot T, Hudis CA, et al. The role of bevacizumab in solid tumours: A literature based meta-analysis of randomised trials. Eur J Cancer 2017;75:245–58.

31. Rini BI, Powles T, Atkins MB, et al. Atezolizumab plus bevacizumab versus sunitinib in patients with previously untreated metastatic renal cell carcinoma (IMmotion151): a multicentre, open-label, phase 3, randomised controlled trial. Lancet 2019; 393(10189):2404–15.

32. Choueiri TK, Escudier B, Powles T, et al. Cabozantinib versus everolimus in advanced renal cell carcinoma (METEOR): final results from a randomised, open-label, phase 3 trial. Lancet Oncol 2016;17(7): 917–27.

33. Bracarda S, Bamias A, Casper J, et al. Is axitinib still a valid option for mrcc in the second-line setting? prognostic factor analyses from the AXIS trial. Clin Genitourin Cancer 2019;17(3):e689–703.

34. Rankin EB, Fuh KC, Castellini L, et al. Direct regulation of GAS6/AXL signaling by HIF promotes renal metastasis through SRC and MET. Proc Natl Acad Sci U S A 2014;111(37):13373–8.

35. Nadal RM, MA, Stein M, , et. al. Results of Phase I Plus Expansion Cohorts of Cabozantinib Plus Nivolumab and Cabozantinib/nivolumab Plus Ipilimumab In Patients With Metastatic Urothelial Carcinoma And Other Genitourinary Malignancies. ASCO GU 2018; 2018; San Francisco, CA.

36. Choueiri TK, Apolo AB, Powles T, et al. A phase 3, randomized, open-label study of nivolumab combined with cabozantinib vs sunitinib in patients with previously untreated advanced or metastatic renal cell carcinoma (RCC; CheckMate 9ER). J Clin Oncol 2018;36(15_suppl): TPS4598.

37. Blinman PL, Davis ID, Martin A, et al. Patients' preferences for adjuvant sorafenib after resection of renal cell carcinoma in the SORCE trial: what makes it worthwhile? Ann Oncol 2018;29(2):370–6.

38. Motzer RJ, Haas NB, Donskov F, et al. Randomized phase III trial of adjuvant pazopanib versus placebo after nephrectomy in patients with localized or locally advanced renal cell carcinoma. J Clin Oncol 2017;35(35):3916–23.

39. Staehler M, Motzer RJ, George DJ, et al. Adjuvant sunitinib in patients with high-risk renal cell

carcinoma: safety, therapy management, and patient-reported outcomes in the S-TRAC trial. Ann Oncol 2018;29(10):2098–104.

40. LaFleur MW, Muroyama Y, Drake CG, et al. Inhibitors of the PD-1 pathway in tumor therapy. J Immunol 2018;200(2):375–83.

41. Balar AV, Galsky MD, Rosenberg JE, et al. Atezolizumab as first-line treatment in cisplatin-ineligible patients with locally advanced and metastatic urothelial carcinoma: a single-arm, multicentre, phase 2 trial. Lancet 2017;389(10064): 67–76.

42. Uzzo R, Bex A, Rini BI, et al. A phase III study of atezolizumab (atezo) vs placebo as adjuvant therapy in renal cell carcinoma (RCC) patients (pts) at high risk of recurrence following resection (IMmotion010). J Clin Oncol 2017;35(15_suppl):TPS4598.

43. Choueiri TK, Quinn DI, Zhang T, et al. KEYNOTE-564: A phase 3, randomized, double blind, trial of pembrolizumab in the adjuvant treatment of renal cell carcinoma. J Clin Oncol 2018;36(15_suppl): TPS4599.

44. Bex A, Grünwald V, Russo P, et al. 927TiP - A phase III, randomized, placebo-controlled trial of adjuvant nivolumab plus ipilimumab in patients (pts) with localized renal cell carcinoma (RCC) who are at high risk of relapse after radical or partial nephrectomy (CheckMate 914). Ann Oncol 2018;29:viii330.

45. Tarhini AA, Edington H, Butterfield LH, et al. Immune monitoring of the circulation and the tumor microenvironment in patients with regionally advanced melanoma receiving neoadjuvant ipilimumab. PLoS One 2014;9(2):e87705.

46. Najjar YG, Rayman P, Jia X, et al. Myeloid-derived suppressor cell subset accumulation in renal cell carcinoma parenchyma is associated with intratumoral expression of IL1β, IL8, CXCL5, and Mip-1α. Clin Cancer Res 2017;23(9):2346–55.

47. Aggen DH, Ghasemzadeh A, Mao W, et al. Preclinical development of combination therapy targeting the dominant cytokine interleukin-1β for renal cell carcinoma. J Clin Oncol 2019;37(15_suppl):e14237.

48. Alt AL, Boorjian SA, Lohse CM, et al. Survival after complete surgical resection of multiple metastases from renal cell carcinoma. Cancer 2011;117(13): 2873–82.

49. Méjean A, Ravaud A, Thezenas S, et al. Sunitinib alone or after nephrectomy in metastatic renal-cell carcinoma. N Engl J Med 2018;379(5):417–27.

50. Drake CG, Stein MN. The immunobiology of kidney cancer. J Clin Oncol 2018;36(36):3547–52.

51. McDermott DF, Cheng S-C, Signoretti S, et al. The high-dose aldesleukin "select" trial: a trial to prospectively validate predictive models of response to treatment in patients with metastatic renal cell carcinoma. Clin Cancer Res 2015;21(3):561–8.

52. Papadimitrakopoulou V, Tannir N, Bernatchez C, et al. P2. 07-062 PIVOT-02: Phase 1/2 study of NKTR-214 and nivolumab in patients with locally advanced or metastatic solid tumor malignancies. J Thorac Oncol 2017;12(11):S2153.

53. Antonioli L, Blandizzi C, Pacher P, et al. Immunity, inflammation and cancer: a leading role for adenosine. Nat Rev Cancer 2013;13(12):842–57.

54. Motzer RJ, LC-H, Emamekhoo H, et al. ENTRATA: Randomized, double-blind, phase 2 study of telaglenastat (tela; CB-839) + everolimus (E) vs. placebo (pbo) + E in patients (pts) with advanced/metastatic renal cell carcinoma (mRCC). ESMO 2019; 2019; Barcelona, Spain.

55. Jonasch E, Park EK, Thamake S, et al. An open-label phase II study to evaluate PT2977 for the treatment of von Hippel-Lindau disease-associated renal cell carcinoma. J Clin Oncol 2019;37(7_suppl):TPS680.

56. 2019 E. ESMO 2019: A First-in-Human Phase 1/2 Trial of the Oral HIF-2a Inhibitor PT2977 in Patients with Advanced RCC. 2019. Available at: https://www.urotoday.com/conference-highlights/esmo-2019/esmo-2019-kidney-cancer/115345-esmo-2019-a-first-in-human-phase-1-2-trial-of-the-oral-hif-2a-inhibitor-pt2977-in-patients-with-advanced-rcc.html. Accessed June 21, 2020.

Harnessing Natural Killer Cell Function for Genitourinary Cancers

Nina Bhardwaj, MD, PhD[a],*, Adam M. Farkas, PhD[b,1], Zeynep Gul, MD[c,1], John P. Sfakianos, MD[d]

KEYWORDS

- Natural killer cells • NK cells • Bladder cancer • Renal cancer • RCC • Genitourinary cancer
- Immunotherapy

KEY POINTS

- Recent studies show that urologic tumors are infiltrated by natural killer (NK) cells and that these NK cells are often dysfunctional.
- Strategies interfering with inhibitory axes have significant potential to alleviate this dysfunction.
- Preclinical studies show that NK-cell antitumor functions can be enhanced.
- Diverse, NK cell–centric clinical trials are ongoing for patients with genitourinary cancers.

BACKGROUND

Natural killer (NK cells) are cytotoxic lymphocytes that are members of the innate immune system. As such, they lack the antigen specificity of T and B cells but recognize cells that have downregulated human leukocyte antigen (HLA) class I and upregulated markers of cell stress, such as MICA, MICB, ULBP-1, and the polio virus receptor. Because loss of class I and expression of these stress ligands often occurs during viral infection and cancer, NK cells are important components of both antiviral defense and tumor immunosurveillance. NK-cell recognition of potential target cells relies on the ability to detect missing self, as initially proposed by Klause Kärre.[1] During surveillance in the peripheral blood, secondary lymphoid organs, and tissue, killer immunoglobulinlike receptors (KIRs) on NK cells recognize HLA-A, HLA-B, and HLA-C expressed

by putative targets. Binding of the KIR to its cognate class I HLA molecule delivers an inhibitory signal to the NK cell via phosphorylation of ITIM (immunoreceptor tyrosine-based inhibitory motif) motifs in the KIR's cytosolic domain (**Fig. 1**, top). Subsequent recruitment of the SHP-1 tyrosine phosphatase results in suppression of NK-cell effector function and prevents the NK cell from killing the target. However, when an NK cell encounters a virally infected cell or tumor cell that has downregulated class I HLA, the inhibitory KIR-HLA signal is not delivered. If there is a concurrent, activating signal delivered through interaction of a cell stress ligand with its cognate, activating receptor on the NK cell, then NK effector functions can proceed (see **Fig. 1**, bottom).

NK cells perform 4 major effector functions after successful recognition of target cells (see **Fig. 1**, bottom). The first is direct cytolytic activity resulting in specific killing of the target through the

---

[a] Department of Hematology & Oncology, Icahn School of Medicine at Mount Sinai, The Tisch Cancer Institute, Hess CSM Building 1470 Madison Avenue, New York, NY 10029, USA; [b] Department of Hematology & Oncology, Icahn School of Medicine at Mount Sinai, The Tisch Cancer Institute, 1470 Madison Avenue, New York, NY 10029, USA; [c] Department of Urology, Icahn School of Medicine at Mount Sinai, Icahn Building, 1425 Madison Avenue, New York, NY 10029, USA; [d] Department of Urology, Icahn School of Medicine at Mount Sinai, 1 Gustave L. Levy Place, Box 1272, New York, NY 10029, USA

[1] Equal Contribution

* Corresponding author.

E-mail address: Nina.Bhardwaj@mssm.edu

Urol Clin N Am 47 (2020) 433–442
https://doi.org/10.1016/j.ucl.2020.07.002

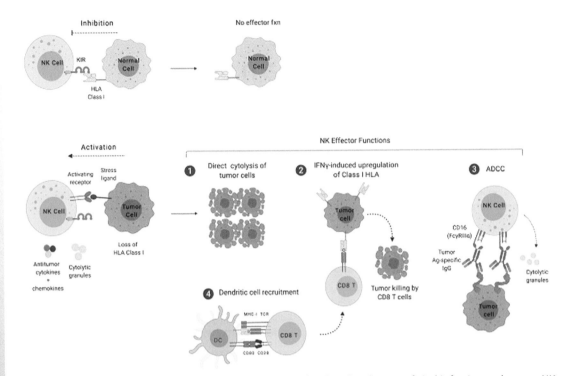

Fig. 1. Target recognition and effector functions of NK cells. (*Top*) In the absence of viral infection and cancer, NK cells receive inhibitory signals through class I HLA-KIR interactions. (*Bottom*) Cells that have lost class I HLA expression and upregulated molecules associated with cell stress deliver stimulatory signals to NK cells, resulting in the execution of effector function. The major antitumor functions of NK cells include production of tumoricidal cytokines, direct cytolytic activity, recruitment of dendritic cells (DCs), and antibody-dependent cellular cytotoxicity (ADCC). Ag, antigen; CD, cluster of differentiation; fxn, function; IFN, interferon; Ig, immunoglobulin; MHC, major histocompatibility complex; TCR, time to castration resistance.

induction of apoptosis. NK cells, unlike naive CD8$^+$ T cell, contain preformed, cytolytic granules that are released into the synapse between the NK cell and target cell as the NK cell degranulates. These granules contain perforin, a protein that creates holes in the target cell membrane, and various granzymes: serine proteases that cleave caspases in the target cell, thus initiating an apoptotic cascade. The second NK-cell effector function is the release of cytokines with both tumoricidal and chemoattractant properties. Two of the best-characterized NK-cell cytokines are interferon (IFN-γ) and tumor necrosis factor (TNF-α) IFN-γ promotes upregulation of class I HLA by target cells. Although this generally renders the targets less susceptible to NK cell–mediated killing, it is important for the concurrent or subsequent CD8$^+$ T cell response by facilitating presentation of peptides loaded on class I HLA to specific CD8$^+$ T cell clones. TNF-α has direct tumoricidal effects on binding TNF receptor 1 (TNFR1), and also plays important roles in monocyte/macrophage function, and destabilization of regulatory T cells.[2] More recently, a third NK-cell effector

function has been identified pertaining to the recruitment of dendritic cells (DCs). NK cells have been shown to produce the DC chemoattractant cytokines XCL1, XCL2, and CCL5, as well as the DC growth factor FLT3 ligand.[3] These cytokines can recruit DC to tumor-draining lymph nodes and tumor tissue itself, thereby improving antigen presentation to tumor-reactive T cells. In addition, a fourth NK-cell effector function is antibody-dependent cellular cytotoxicity (ADCC). During ADCC, CD16, a receptor that binds the Fc region of immunoglobulin G1, is cross-linked by antibodies bound to extracellular proteins on tumor cells. This cross-linking induces a conformational change in the signaling domains of CD16 leading to phosphorylation of its associated ITAM (immunoreceptor tyrosine-based activating motif), and a subsequent signaling cascade that results in NK-cell degranulation, and lysis of the antibody-coated target cell.[4]

Two major subpopulations of NK cells have been identified in humans: CD56^{bright} and CD56^{dim}CD16$^+$. CD56^{bright} NK cells are considered developmentally less mature but secrete most of the cytokines discussed earlier. CD56^{dim}CD16$^+$ NK cells represent more mature NK cells, and possess more potent cytolytic capability compared with the CD56^{bright} subset. Approximately 10% of healthy peripheral blood mononuclear cells (PBMCs) are NK cells, and, of these ~5% to 10% are CD56^{bright} with the remaining cells belonging to the CD56^{dim}CD16$^+$ subpopulation. However, patients with prostate cancer, and non–muscle-invasive (NMI) bladder cancer (BlCa), have increased frequencies of circulating NK cells,[5,6] suggesting that genitourinary tumors can elicit an immune response in the periphery. Furthermore, infiltration of CD56^{bright} NK cells has been associated with improved survival in both BlCa and renal cell carcinoma (RCC).[7–9]

As mentioned earlier, unlike T cells, NK cells do not recognize specific peptide antigens, and instead detect the presence or absence of class I HLA. However, loss of HLA in the presence of additional inhibitory signals elicits a suboptimal effector response, whereas HLA expression in the context of strong activating signals can elicit a strong response.[10] The magnitude of NK-cell functional responses is calibrated by integrating stimulatory and inhibitory signals delivered through a diverse array of accessory receptors. Three such inhibitory receptors, NKG2A, Tim-3, and TIGIT (T-cell immunoreceptor with immunoglobulin and ITIM domains), are expressed by NK cells in solid tumors (**Fig. 2**), with Tim-3 expression reported as anticorrelated with survival in patients with BlCa.[11–14] When NKG2A binds its ligand, the noncanonical class I molecule HLA-E expressed on tumor cells, phosphorylation of its cytosolic ITIM occurs, followed by recruitment of the SHP-1 phosphatase. SHP-1 can then prevent phosphorylation of the stimulatory motifs associated with neighboring activating

receptors.[15] This process ultimately results in suppression of NK-cell effector functions. Tim-3 binds multiple ligands expressed on both tumor cells and immune cells, including soluble galectin-9 and HMGB1, phosphatidylserine on apoptotic cells, and CEACAM-1.[16] Unlike many other inhibitory receptors, Tim-3 does not contain an ITIM motif but uses the adaptor protein Bat3 to mediate suppression of NK-cell function. In addition, TIGIT mediates NK-cell inhibition via canonical ITIM signaling like NKG2A; however, it shares the ligands CD112 and CD155 with the activating receptor DNAM-1 (CD226). This competition to bind shared ligands provides another layer of control in tuning the NK-cell response. The inhibitory receptor programmed cell death protein 1 (PD-1), although highly relevant in the context of immune checkpoint blockade (ICB) therapy, is predominantly expressed by tumor-resident T cells, with minimal expression by NK cells.

NATURAL KILLER CELLS IN BLADDER CANCER
Natural Killer Cells Infiltrate Bladder Tumors

Most studies of tumor-infiltrating lymphocytes (TILs) in BlCa have focused on T cells, with much recent attention appropriately focused on the role of the PD-1–programmed death-ligand 1 inhibitory axis, and ICB approaches to ameliorate it.[17–19] However, a recent study profiling 50 NMI and muscle-invasive (MI) bladder tumors suggests that ~25% of the immune infiltrate is made up of NK cells, making them the most frequent lineage examined.[7] In addition, despite this small cohort, a statistically significant correlation was found between the frequency of CD56^{bright} NK cells and overall survival (OS).[7] Importantly, in healthy bladder,[20,21] and in noninvolved bladder tissue

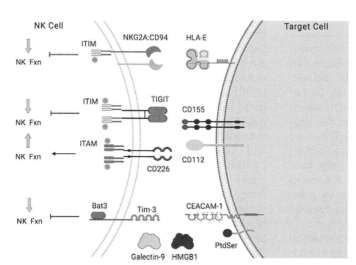

Fig. 2. Inhibitory receptors tune the magnitude of NK cell effector function. Expression of inhibitory receptors expressed by NK cells in solid tumors. The ligands for each receptor are shown on the right, and the effect on NK cell effector function shown on the left. ITAM, immunoreceptor tyrosine-based activating motif.

from cystectomy specimens (Farkas, 2020; unpublished observations), NK cells represent a much smaller component of the resident immune cells. This finding suggests that NK cells can specifically infiltrate and conduct immunosurveillance of bladder tumors, making them rational targets for immunotherapeutic modulation.

Natural Killer Cell Function in the Tumor and Peripheral Blood of Patients with Bladder Cancer

Immune exhaustion occurs during chronic infection as well as cancer, and refers to defects in effector functions that result from prolonged stimulation and suppressive factors in the tumor microenvironment (TME).[22] Few studies have examined the functional potential of tumor-resident NK cells, in part because of challenges associated with establishing a pipeline in which a sufficient quantity of freshly resected tumor tissue is processed and analyzed in the research laboratory. Similarly, there are few data comparing differences in NK-cell function between patient-matched peripheral blood and tumor. An early study found no defect in the ability of peripheral blood NK cells from patients with BlCa to degranulate in response to HLA-deficient target cells compared with healthy donors. However, there was a substantial defect in degranulation observed in NK cells isolated from tumor and lymph node.[5] In contrast, subsequent work showed that the peripheral blood NK cells from patients with NMI BlCa had no cytolytic defect, whereas those from patients with MI disease did.[23] In addition, a recent study found that tumor-resident CD56[bright] NK cells produced more IFN-γ than CD56[dim]CD16[+] cells, but did not compare these cells with NK cells in healthy or patient blood.[7]

The Role of Natural Killer Cells in Bladder Cancer Treatments

Bacillus Calmette-Guérin (BCG) was the first immunotherapy widely used for cancer treatment, but its precise mechanism of efficacy is not defined. Several studies have pointed toward a role for NK cells in BCG responders. A study of healthy volunteers receiving BCG vaccination showed that production of interleukin (IL)-1b, IL-6, and TNF-α by NK cells was enhanced during ex vivo restimulation after vaccination, suggesting that NK cells from BCG-experienced individuals develop a form of memory.[24] In addition, NK cells cultured in the presence of BCG for 1 week gained improved cytolytic function against bladder tumor cell lines.[25]

Novel, preclinical studies have also focused on improving NK-cell surveillance against bladder tumors. Combination chemotherapy–epigenetic therapy using cisplatin and an EZH2 inhibitor showed efficacy against MI BlCa, both in direct tumor killing and in improving the NK-cell response against surviving tumor clones.[26] NK cells can be differentiated in vitro from cord blood–derived progenitors, and it is possible to activate NK cells isolated from adult peripheral blood with cytokines such as IL-2, IL-15, IL-12, IL-18, and IL-21, all of which improve effector functionality, induce proliferation, and improve NK-cell survival[27] (**Fig. 3**). Both of these approaches can be used as sources of NK cells for adoptive cell transfer therapy. For example, adoptive transfer of IL-2/IL-15–activated NK cells from healthy donors into immunodeficient mice bearing orthotopic, chemoresistant bladder tumors resulted in tumor regression. However, transfer of activated NK cells isolated from patients with high-grade NMI BlCa was less effective, suggesting that peripheral blood NK cells from patients with BlCa are exhausted.[28] In addition, preclinical ICB to enhance NK-cell tumor surveillance in murine models and primary human cells ex vivo, although not exclusively in BlCa, have shown that blockade of Tim-3,[29,30] TIGIT,[13] and NKG2A[11] all improve NK function.

Clinical Trials Targeting Natural Killer Cells in Bladder Cancer

Many ongoing and recently completed trials of NK cell–centric immunotherapy involve adoptive transfer of in vitro differentiated NK cells, infusion of preactivated adult NK cells, or transfer of NK cells stably transduced with chimeric antigen receptor (CAR) T cell--like receptors that confer tumor-antigen specificity (see **Fig. 3**). Most of these studies use haploidentical donors for source material, and are infused into patients with hematologic malignancies such as chronic myeloid leukemia, acute myeloid leukemia, chronic lymphocytic leukemia, and non-Hodgkin lymphoma.[27,31] However, there are also NK cell–centric trials for patients with metastatic, locally advanced, and/or cisplatin-ineligible BlCa. For example, there is a phase I/II dose-escalation study of DF1001, a novel biologic that simultaneously targets Her2[+] tumors and activates NK cells (NCT04143711). This study will enroll 220 patients with solid tumors, including those with metastatic and locally advanced BlCa, and includes a DF1001+X-PD-1 arm. Several trials will also determine the effects of cytokine activation on NK-cell efficacy in BlCa, such as a phase II study of 205 patients with cisplatin-ineligible MI BlCa who will receive bempegaldesleukin, a PEGylated IL-2, alone or in combination with X-PD-1 (NCT03785925). Two trials being conducted in China are testing the efficacy of so-called

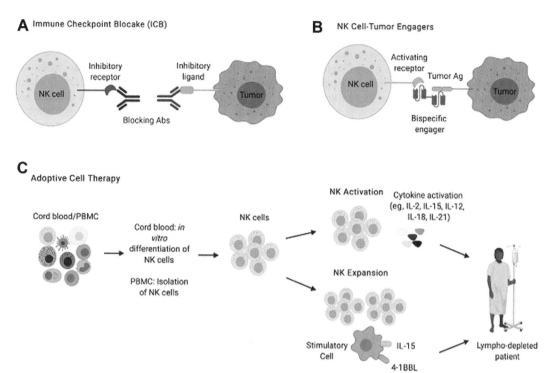

Fig. 3. Major approaches to NK cell immunotherapy: 3 broad immunotherapeutic strategies to improve NK cell tumor surveillance currently used preclinically and in clinical trials. (*A*) ICB relies on the administration of monoclonal antibodies that prevent signaling through inhibitory receptors. (*B*) NK-tumor engagers are biologics with double or triple specificities. These molecules confer specificity to NK-tumor interactions by binding a protein antigen expressed by tumor cells and simultaneously delivering a stimulatory signal to the NK cell through an activating or cytokine receptor. (*C*) Adoptive cell therapy approaches infuse NK cells isolated from PBMCs, or differentiated in vitro from cord blood progenitors, into autologous, haploidentical, or allogeneic recipients. The transferred NK cells can be preactivated with cytokines to enhance NK cell effector functions or can be expanded using irradiated stimulatory cells engineered to express cytokines and stimulatory ligands. Ab, antibody.

cytokine-induced killer (CIK) cells; autologous PBMCs expanded and activated to enhance NK and T cell function. One of these will examine infusion of CIK cells or CIK cells plus chemotherapy in individuals with MI BICa (NCT02489890). The second will test infusions of autologous PBMC after culture conditions intended to increase the number and activity of NK and T cells, as well as dendritic cells (D-CIK) using IL-2, IFN-γ, IL-1α, X-CD3, and X-PD-1 (NCT02886897), In addition, a phase Ib neoadjuvant trial in patients with MI BICa before scheduled, radical cystectomy will compare X-PD-1 treatment with a combination of X-PD-1 and lirilumab (NCT03532451). Lirilumab is monoclonal antibody that blocks the interaction of 3 inhibitory KIRs (KIR2DL1/2/3) with various HLA-C alleles, with the goal of decreasing the inhibitory interactions that might preclude optimal NK-cell function.

NATURAL KILLER CELLS IN KIDNEY CANCER

In RCC, NK cells represent a significant portion of TILs.[32] In a rat model of RCC, injection of an NK cell–depleting antibody significantly increased the tumor growth rate, suggesting that NK cells are important in antitumor defense.[33] Eckl and colleagues[8] showed that, after stratifying patients into 2 groups based on the percentage of their TILs that were NK cells, patients with more NK cells had significantly longer cancer-specific survival. Another study found that, as the tumor T stage increased, the percentage of infiltrating NK cells decreased significantly.[34]

Natural Killer Cell Function in the Tumor and Peripheral Blood of Patients with Renal Cell Carcinoma

Studies have identified pathways by which the TME inhibits NK-cell function. Prinz and colleagues[35] found that a significantly lower number of NK cells in TIL expressed perforin or granzyme B than NK cells from the nontumor kidney. In addition, TIL NK cells had low levels of phosphorylated ERK1/2 (extracellular signal-regulated kinase) and JNK (Jun kinase), which are required to initiate lytic granule exocytosis. ERK activation depends on diacylglycerol, which is metabolized by diacylglycerol kinase (DGK). DGK levels were higher in TIL NK cells than in normal renal tissue, leading to less ERK activation and poor NK-cell degranulation. In addition, DGK inhibition led to improved NK-cell cytotoxicity. These findings suggest that DGK and suppression of the ERK pathway may be a way for RCC cells to escape NK cell–mediated destruction.[35] Xia and colleagues[36] showed that exosomes from RCC tumor cells inhibited NK-cell activity in a dose-dependent manner. They then showed that the exosomes of patients with RCC expressed increased levels of transforming growth factor (TGF) β-1 and that inhibiting TGFβ-1 improved NK-cell cytotoxic acitivity.[36]

The Role of Natural Killer Cells in Renal Cell Carcinoma Treatments

There are several medications approved for the treatment of RCC, many of which affect NK-cell activity. IL-2 was the first widely used treatment of advanced RCC and is the only medical treatment that has resulted in a cure. In the 1980s, scientists showed that IL-2 increases NK-cell cytotoxicity.[37] In addition, in patients with metastatic RCC treated with IL-2 plus or minus IFNα and histamine, low intratumoral CD57[+] NK-cell count was an independent poor prognostic factor (<50 cells/mm^2 tumor tissue; hazard ratio, 2.1; P = .01). These findings show that at least some of the antitumor activity of IL-2 is through NK-cell cytotoxicity. Sunitinib and sorafenib are multikinase inhibitors with antiangiogenic effects. Studies have shown that sorafenib but not sunitinib significantly reduced NK-cell activity, possibly through suppressing the ERK pathway.[38,39] Axitinib has been shown to exert its antitumor effects at least partially through increasing RCC tumor susceptibility to NK cell–mediated degranulation.[40]

Clinical Trials Targeting Natural Killer Cells in Renal Cell Carcinoma

Although NK cells do not express PD-1 to the extent that T cells do, there is an active clinical trial to determine the effects of nivolumab on NK-cell function and cytotoxicity in both the blood and tumor tissue in patients with metastatic RCC (NCT03891485). Most other clinical trials, as in BICa, involve adoptive transfer of in vitro differentiated NK cells or infusion of preactivated adult NK cells. For example, there is currently a trial underway to determine whether there are any differences in progression-free survival (PFS) between patients treated with the PD-1 inhibitor camrelizumab alone or in combination with CIK in patients with metastatic RCC who have progressed on tyrosine kinase inhibitors (NCT03987698). There are several trials that include incubating CIK cells with DCs. Coculture of DCs and CIKs (D-CIKs) improves CIK cell antitumor activity through cell-to-cell contact by increasing NK-cell proliferation and cytotoxicity. One phase II trial is assessing the effect of a PD-1 inhibitor and D-CIK on PFS (NCT02886897) and another is assessing the effect of axitinib in combination with D-CIKs and the PD-1 inhibitor pembrolizumab on PFS (NCT03736330). Alternatively, DCs can be pulsed with tumor lysates or tumor-associated antigens to create a DC vaccine. A study is underway to compare outcomes of DC vaccines and CIKs compared with IL-2/IFNα in patients with RCC (NCT00862303).

NATURAL KILLER CELLS IN PROSTATE CANCER

Although, compared with bladder and kidney cancer, prostate cancer is considered less immunogenic, NK cells have been identified in prostate cancer tumors.[41] In both tumor and healthy prostatic tissue, infiltrating NK cells expressed activation markers but had poor degranulation capabilities compared with circulating NK cells. When comparing NK cells found in tumor with those in healthy tissue, expression of the activating receptors NKp46 and NKG2D was significantly decreased and the inhibitory receptor ILT2 was significantly increased. In addition, decreased expression of NKp46 and NKG2D and increased expression of ILT2 were more pronounced in NK cells from metastatic tumors than from localized or locoregional tumors (ie, tumor with extraprostatic extension, seminal vesicle invasion, or local lymph node invasion).[42]

NK-cell activity has been correlated with prostate cancer outcomes. Increased concentrations of infiltrating NK cells have been associated with a lower risk of cancer progression.[43] When examining circulating NK cells, low levels of NK activity have been associated with an increased likelihood of having a positive prostate biopsy.[41,44,45] Koo and colleagues[46] found that patients with prostate cancer had a significantly higher CD56[dim]/CD56[bright] cell ratio compared with controls (41.8 vs 30.3; P<.001) and that the ratio gradually increased as disease stage progressed (P for trend = .001). They also showed that levels of NK-cell activity were significantly lower in patients with prostate cancer than in controls, and patients with higher-stage disease had a greater reduction of activity.[46] Another study found that, among patients with metastatic prostate cancer, blood levels of the activating receptors NKp30 and NKp46 were predictive of OS and time to castration resistance (TCR) (OS, P = .0018 and .0009; TCR, P = .007 and P<.0001 respectively).[42] There is currently a clinical trial underway to prospectively validate these findings (NCT02963155).

Several studies have also examined how the prostate cancer TME inhibits or evades NK cells. TGFβ has been identified in the prostate cancer microenvironment and is known to inhibit NK-cell function. In addition, in coculture experiments, prostate cancer cells promoted the expression of the inhibitory receptor ILT2 and suppressed the expression of activating receptors NKp46, NKG2D, and CD16, preventing NK-cell activity against tumor cells.[47] As in BICa, exosomes play a critical role in prostate cancer's ability to invade the immune response. Lundholm and colleagues[48] showed that prostate cancer cells secrete exosomes, which downregulate NKG2D expression, leading to impaired cytotoxicity in vitro. As expected from these results, patients with castration-resistant prostate cancer had a significant decrease in the expression of NKG2D on circulating NK cells compared with controls.[48]

The Role of Natural Killer Cells in Prostate Cancer Treatments

The effects of current prostate cancer therapies on NK cells are not well defined and research on the issue is limited. Studies to determine whether androgen deprivation leads to an increase in NK-cell tumor infiltration have mixed results.[43,49] At present, sipuleucel-T is the only immunotherapy approved to treat prostate cancer. Sipuleucel-T is generated by culturing autologous blood mononuclear cells with a fusion protein composed of prostatic acid phosphatase and granulocyte-macrophage colony-stimulating factor. The final product is composed primary of T cells but also contains NK cells.[50] To better understand the effects of sipuleucel-T on the TME, a trial was performed in which patients with localized prostate cancer were treated with sipuleucel-T as a neoadjuvant. After radical prostatectomy (RP), TILs in the specimen were assessed and compared with the infiltrating immune cells in the pretreatment prostate biopsy specimens. NK-cell levels were not higher in RP specimens, indicating that NK cells do not play a significant role in sipuleucel-T activity.[51]

Clinical Trials Targeting Natural Killer Cells in Prostate Cancer

Immunotherapy as a treatment of prostate cancer has not been as well explored as in renal cancer

and BICa. Therefore, there are currently several studies underway to evaluating the effects of various treatments on NK-cell activity. For example, there is a phase 1 clinical trial assessing the effects of intraprostatic injection of mobilan, which is an adenovirus carrying TLR5 (toll-like receptor 5) and a TLR5 activator, on circulating immune-cell levels in patients with prostate cancer, including NK-cell counts (NCT02654938). At Johns Hopkins, a clinical trial is underway to assess the effect of neoadjuvant enoblituzumab, an antibody directed against cancer stem cells, on the intraprostatic immune response, including mean NK-cell density, after RP (NCT02923180). At Henry Ford, a study of intraprostatic injections of an adenovirus carrying IL-12 in patients with recurrence after brachytherapy is currently underway. Outcomes of interest include the association with disease-specific outcomes, such as prostate-specific antigen response and disease-free survival with serum NK-cell cytolytic activity (NCT02555397). Roswell Park Cancer Institute is currently performing a study to determine whether radiation therapy potentiates the effects of sipuleucel-T in patients with bone metastasis. One of the primary end points will be the quantification of circulating NK cells (NCT01833208). There is also a trial that involves transfer of autologous NK cells and the protease inhibitor bortezomib, which has been shown to increase the sensitivity of cancer cells to NK-cell activity[52] in patients with metastatic prostate cancer (NCT00720785).

SUMMARY

NK cells recognize target cells that have downregulated HLA class I and upregulated markers of cell stress. These changes often occur during viral infections and cancer and therefore NK cells play an important role in the body's defense against these disease processes. The magnitude of NK cell's functional response is determined by integrating stimulatory and inhibitory signals delivered though an array of receptors on the NK cell. NK cells infiltrate bladder, kidney, and prostate tumors. In all 3 malignancies, the frequency of NK cells in tumor tissue has been correlated with survival. There are currently several trials designed to increase NK-cell activity to improve cancer outcomes.

CLINICAL CARE POINTS

- When an NK cell encounters a potential target cell there are 2 possible outcomes.

- ○ Inhibition: KIRs on NK cells recognize HLA class 1. Binding of the KIR to its cognate class I HLA molecule delivers an inhibitory signal to the NK cell and prevents the cell from killing its target.
  - ○ Activation: when an NK cell encounters a tumor cell that has downregulated class I HLA, an inhibitory signal is not delivered.
- Magnitude of NK-cell activity depends on the stimulation of several accessory receptors found on NK cells.
- NK cells have been found in bladder, kidney, and prostate tumor tissue.
- In all 3 malignancies, higher NK-cell levels are associated with better outcomes.
- Blockade of inhibitory NK-cell receptors (such as Tim-3) have been shown, in preclinical models and in ex vivo human cells, to improve NK-cell function and may serve as future drug targets.
- NK cells likely play a greater role in cancer immunotherapies than previously realized. For example, IL-2, which was the first immunotherapy for RCC and the only one that has led to durable cures, is a potent NK-cell activator.
- Several trials are underway to determine how to best activate NK cells.
- At present there are many clinical trials that involve adoptive transfer of preactivated NK cells.

DISCLOSURE

This work was funded by a Translational Team Science Award from the Department of Defense (CA181008) to N. Bhardwaj and J.P. Sfakianos, and National Institutes of Health R01 CA201189 to N. Bhardwaj. N. Bhardwaj is an advisory board member for Neon, Tempest, CPS Companion Diagnostics, Curevac, Primevax, Novartis, Array BioPharma, Roche, Avidea, Boehringer Ingelheim, Rome Therapeutics, and Roswell Park. N. Bhardwaj is an extramural member of the Parker Institute for Cancer Immunotherapy, and has received research support from Celldex, Genentech, Oncovir, and Regeneron. A.M. Farkas, Z. Gul, and J.P. Sfakianos have no disclosures to report.

REFERENCES

1. Kärre K. NK cells, MHC class I molecules and the missing self. Scand J Immunol 2002;55(3):221–8.
2. Balkwill F. Tumour necrosis factor and cancer. Nat Rev Cancer 2009;9(5):361–71.
3. Kevin C. Barry, Joy Hsu, Miranda L. Broz, et al. A natural killer–dendritic cell axis defines checkpoint therapy–responsive tumor microenvironments. Nature Medicine volume 24, p:1178–1191(2018).
4. Gómez Román VR, Murray JC, Weiner LM. Chapter 1 - antibody-dependent cellular cytotoxicity (ADCC). In: Ackerman ME, Nimmerjahn F, editors. Antibody Fc. Boston: Academic Press; 2014. p. 1–27.
5. Tsujihashi H, Matsuda H, Uejima S, et al. Role of natural killer cells in bladder tumor. Eur Urol 1989;16(6):444–9.
6. Audenet F, Farkas AM, Anastos H, et al. Immune phenotype of peripheral blood mononuclear cells in patients with high-risk non-muscle invasive bladder cancer. World J Urol 2018;36(11):1741–8.
7. Mukherjee N, Ji N, Hurez V, et al. Intratumoral CD56(bright) natural killer cells are associated with improved survival in bladder cancer. Oncotarget 2018;9(92):36492–502.
8. Eckl J, Buchner A, Prinz PU, et al. Transcript signature predicts tissue NK cell content and defines renal cell carcinoma subgroups independent of TNM staging. J Mol Med (Berl) 2012;90(1):55–66.
9. Schleypen JS, Baur N, Kammerer R, et al. Cytotoxic markers and frequency predict functional capacity of natural killer cells infiltrating renal cell carcinoma. Clin Cancer Res 2006;12(3 Pt 1):718–25.
10. Morvan MG, Lanier LL. NK cells and cancer: you can teach innate cells new tricks. Nat Rev Cancer 2016;16(1):7–19.
11. Andre P, Denis C, Soulas C, et al. Anti-NKG2A mAb is a checkpoint inhibitor that promotes anti-tumor immunity by unleashing both t and nk cells. Cell 2018;175(7):1731–43.e3.
12. Yang M, Yu Q, Liu J, et al. T-cell immunoglobulin mucin-3 expression in bladder urothelial carcinoma: clinicopathologic correlations and association with survival. J Surg Oncol 2015;112(4):430–5.
13. Zhang Q, Bi J, Zheng X, et al. Blockade of the checkpoint receptor TIGIT prevents NK cell exhaustion and elicits potent anti-tumor immunity. Nat Immunol 2018;19(7):723–32.
14. Zhang Y, Cai P, Liang T, et al. TIM-3 is a potential prognostic marker for patients with solid tumors: A systematic review and meta-analysis. Oncotarget 2017;8(19):31705–13.
15. Braud VM, Allan DS, O'Callaghan CA, et al. HLA-E binds to natural killer cell receptors CD94/NKG2A, B and C. Nature 1998;391(6669):795–9.
16. Anderson AC, Joller N, Kuchroo VK. Lag-3, Tim-3, and TIGIT: co-inhibitory receptors with specialized functions in immune regulation. Immunity 2016;44(5):989–1004.
17. Rosenberg JE, Hoffman-Censits J, Powles T, et al. Atezolizumab in patients with locally advanced and metastatic urothelial carcinoma who have progressed following treatment with platinum-based chemotherapy: a single-arm, multicentre, phase 2 trial. Lancet 2016;387(10031):1909–20.

18. Wang L, Gong Y, Saci A, et al. Fibroblast growth factor receptor 3 alterations and response to PD-1/PD-L1 blockade in patients with metastatic urothelial cancer. Eur Urol 2019;76(5):599–603.

19. Sharma P, Retz M, Siefker-Radtke A, et al. Nivolumab in metastatic urothelial carcinoma after platinum therapy (CheckMate 275): a multicentre, single-arm, phase 2 trial. Lancet Oncol 2017;18(3):312–22.

20. Yu Z, Liao J, Chen Y, et al. Single-Cell Transcriptomic Map Of The Human And Mouse Bladders. J Am Soc Nephrol 2019;30(11):2159–76.

21. Christmas TJ. Lymphocyte sub-populations in the bladder wall in normal bladder, bacterial cystitis and interstitial cystitis. Br J Urol 1994;73(5):508–15.

22. Wherry EJ, Kurachi M. Molecular and cellular insights into T cell exhaustion. Nat Rev Immunol 2015;15(8):486–99.

23. Carballido J, Alvarez-Mon M, Solovera OJ, et al. Clinical significance of natural killer activity in patients with transitional cell carcinoma of the bladder. J Urol 1990;143(1):29–33.

24. Kleinnijenhuis J, Quintin J, Preijers F, et al. BCG-induced trained immunity in NK cells: Role for non-specific protection to infection. Clin Immunol 2014;155(2):213–9.

25. Garcia-Cuesta EM, Lopez-Cobo S, Alvarez-Maestro M, et al. NKG2D is a Key receptor for recognition of bladder cancer cells by IL-2-activated NK Cells and BCG Promotes NK Cell Activation. Front Immunol 2015;6:284.

26. Ramakrishnan S, Granger V, Rak M, et al. Inhibition of EZH2 induces NK cell-mediated differentiation and death in muscle-invasive bladder cancer. Cell Death Differ 2019;26(10):2100–14.

27. Shimasaki N, Jain A, Campana D. NK cells for cancer immunotherapy. Nat Rev Drug Discov 2020;19(3):200–18.

28. Ferreira-Teixeira M, Paiva-Oliveira D, Parada B, et al. Natural killer cell-based adoptive immunotherapy eradicates and drives differentiation of chemoresistant bladder cancer stem-like cells. BMC Med 2016;14(1):163.

29. da Silva IP, Gallois A, Jimenez-Baranda S, et al. Reversal of NK-cell exhaustion in advanced melanoma by Tim-3 blockade. Cancer Immunol Res 2014;2:410–22.

30. Ndhlovu LC, Lopez-Verges S, Barbour JD, et al. Tim-3 marks human natural killer cell maturation and suppresses cell-mediated cytotoxicity. Blood 2012;119:3734–43. American Society of Hematology.

31. Liu E, Marin D, Banerjee P, et al. Use of CAR-transduced natural killer cells in CD19-positive lymphoid tumors. N Engl J Med 2020;382(6):545–53.

32. Schleypen JS, Von Geldern M, Weiss EH, et al. Renal cell carcinoma-infiltrating natural killer cells express differential repertoires of activating and inhibitory receptors and are inhibited by specific HLA class I allotypes. Int J Cancer 2003;106(6):905–12.

33. Winter BK, Wu S, Nelson AC, et al. Renal cell carcinoma and natural killer cells: studies in a novel rat model in vitro and in vivo. Cancer Res 1992;52(22):6279–86.

34. Cozar JM, Canton J, Tallada M, et al. Analysis of NK cells and chemokine receptors in tumor infiltrating CD4 T lymphocytes in human renal carcinomas. Cancer Immunol Immunother 2005;54(9):858–66.

35. Prinz PU, Mendler AN, Brech D, et al. NK-cell dysfunction in human renal carcinoma reveals diacylglycerol kinase as key regulator and target for therapeutic intervention. Int J Cancer 2014;135(8):1832–41.

36. Xia Y, Zhang Q, Zhen Q, et al. Negative regulation of tumor-infiltrating NK cell in clear cell renal cell carcinoma patients through the exosomal pathway. Oncotarget 2017;8(23):37783–95.

37. Henney CS, Kuribayashi K, Kern DE, et al. Interleukin-2 augments natural killer cell activity. Nature 1981;291(5813):335–8.

38. Krusch M, Salih J, Schlicke M, et al. The kinase inhibitors sunitinib and sorafenib differentially affect NK cell antitumor reactivity in vitro. J Immunol 2009;183(12):8286–94.

39. Manuela S, Matthias K, Baessler T, et al. The kinase inhibitors sunitinib (Sutent®) and Sorafenib (Nexavar®) Differentially Affect Reactivity of NK cells against renal cell cancer. Blood 2007;110(11):4182.

40. Morelli MB, Amantini C, Santoni M, et al. Axitinib induces DNA damage response leading to senescence, mitotic catastrophe, and increased NK cell recognition in human renal carcinoma cells. Oncotarget 2015;6(34):36245–59.

41. Barkin J, Rodriguez-Suarez R, Betito K. Association between natural killer cell activity and prostate cancer: a pilot study. Can J Urol 2017;24(2):8708–13.

42. Pasero C, Gravis G, Granjeaud S, et al. Highly effective NK cells are associated with good prognosis in patients with metastatic prostate cancer. Oncotarget 2015;6(16):14360–73.

43. Gannon PO, Poisson AO, Delvoye N, et al. Characterization of the intra-prostatic immune cell infiltration in androgen-deprived prostate cancer patients. J Immunol Methods 2009;348(1–2):9–17.

44. Tae BS, Jeon BJ, Lee YH, et al. Can natural killer cell activity help screen patients requiring a biopsy for the diagnosis of prostate cancer? Int Braz J Urol 2020;46:244–52.

45. Vidal AC, Howard LE, Wiggins E, et al. Natural killer cell activity and prostate cancer risk in veteran men undergoing prostate biopsy. Cancer Epidemiol 2019;62:101578.

46. Koo KC, Shim DH, Yang CM, et al. Reduction of the CD16(-)CD56bright NK cell subset precedes NK cell dysfunction in prostate cancer. PLoS One 2013;8(11):e78049.

47. Pasero C, Gravis G, Guerin M, et al. Inherent and tumor-driven immune tolerance in the prostate microenvironment impairs natural killer cell antitumor activity. Cancer Res 2016;76(8):2153–65.

48. Lundholm M, Schroder M, Nagaeva O, et al. Prostate tumor-derived exosomes down-regulate NKG2D expression on natural killer cells and CD8+ T cells: mechanism of immune evasion. PLoS One 2014;9(9):e108925.

49. Shen YC, Ghasemzadeh A, Kochel CM, et al. Combining intratumoral Treg depletion with androgen deprivation therapy (ADT): preclinical activity in the Myc-CaP model. Prostate Cancer Prostatic Dis 2018;21(1):113–25.

50. Sheikh NA, Petrylak D, Kantoff PW, et al. Sipuleucel-T immune parameters correlate with survival: an analysis of the randomized phase 3 clinical trials in men with castration-resistant prostate cancer. Cancer Immunol Immunother 2013;62(1):137–47.

51. Fong L, Carroll P, Weinberg V, et al. Activated lymphocyte recruitment into the tumor microenvironment following preoperative sipuleucel-T for localized prostate cancer. J Natl Cancer Inst 2014; 106(11). dju268.

52. Pellom ST Jr, Dudimah DF, Thounaojam MC, et al. Modulatory effects of bortezomib on host immune cell functions. Immunotherapy 2015;7(9):1011–22.

Immunotherapy for Localized Prostate Cancer
The Next Frontier?

Devin Patel, MD[a], Rana McKay, MD[b], J. Kellogg Parsons, MD, MHS[a],*

KEYWORDS

- Immunotherapy • Prostate cancer • Checkpoint inhibitors • PD-L1 • CDK12 • ProstVac-VF
- Sipuleucel-T

KEY POINTS

- Whereas vaccine-based immunotherapy has been promising, other immunotherapy agents, including checkpoint inhibitors, have shown limited efficacy in prostate cancer.
- Ongoing trials of combination therapy and promising biomarkers, including mutations in CDK12, may enhance the efficacy of checkpoint inhibitors for advanced prostate cancer.
- New treatments, including chimeric T lymphocytes and bispecific antibodies, provide future opportunities to enhance the immune response to prostate tumors.

INTRODUCTION

Interactions of the immune system and cancer have been appreciated since the late nineteenth century. Over the past few decades, an increasingly sophisticated understanding of these interactions has driven the development of a novel class of anticancer therapies: immunotherapy. Immunotherapy is the treatment of cancer through suppression or activation of the immune system. Prostate cancer has provided unique opportunities for, and challenges to, immunotherapy drug development.

In this article, we review the mechanisms of the immune response as it relates to cancer biology; outline broad strategies of immunotherapy and key concepts of immunotherapy as it relates to prostate cancer; describe prostate cancer immunotherapy drugs, including pivotal clinical trials and specific indications; and, finally, highlight the emerging role of immunotherapy for localized prostate cancer.

OVERVIEW OF THE IMMUNE RESPONSE AND CANCER
Innate Versus Adaptive Immunity

The immune system relies on an interplay between innate and adaptive immune responses. The innate immune system, which is present at birth and not learned or adapted, includes physical barriers (eg, skin, mucosal barriers), protein barriers (eg, complement components), and cellular barriers. Innate immune cells involved in tumor immunobiology include natural killer cells and macrophages. In addition to creating a nonspecific immune response, innate immune cells are essential for creating the cytokine environment needed for effective antigen presentation to adaptive immune cells. Adaptive immune cells, including cytotoxic CD8[+] lymphocytes and helper Th1/Th2 subclasses of CD4[+] T lymphocytes, rely on antigen presentation to produce a specific immune response.[1] Adaptive immune cells create a specific response to antigens, including tumor antigens. Most of the effort in using the immune

Conflicts of interest: The authors declare no conflicts of interest.
[a] Department of Urology, University of California San Diego, 9400 Campus Point Drive, MC7987, La Jolla, CA 92093, USA; [b] Division of Hematology-Oncology, Department of Internal Medicine, University of California San Diego, La Jolla, CA 92093, USA
* Corresponding author.
E-mail address: k0parsons@ucsd.edu

response for cancer immunobiology has focused on harnessing the adaptive immune response.

Basics of Tumor Immunobiology

Tumor immunobiology is best understood in the context of the cancer immunity cycle. This process starts with release of cancer antigens. Released antigens are then captured and presented by antigen-presenting cells (APCs) to adaptive response T lymphocytes. This process involves the creation of an immune synapse. During first contact between antigen-specific T lymphocytes and an antigen, T lymphocytes are primed. Subsequently the primed cells become activated and differentiate either into effector cells or memory cells. This priming and activation step is dependent on interplay among APCs, T lymphocytes, and stimulatory molecules in the immune microenvironment. T-lymphocyte activation is followed by T-lymphocyte trafficking to tumors through the vascular system and subsequently by T-lymphocyte tumor infiltration through the vascular endothelium into the tissue. Antigen-specific T-cell receptors are then able to recognize cancer cells and lead to cancer cell death. Immune-mediated killing in turn promotes tumor antigen release.

Antigen Release and Presentation

The first step in the cancer immunity cycle is antigen release. Immunogenic tumor cell death, in contrast to apoptotic tumor cell death, leads to necrosis and antigen release. Chemotherapy and radiation therapy also increase antigen release, promoting the framework for combined treatment strategies. Importantly, because of genetic alterations, tumors release neoantigens that are distinguishable from normal counterparts.[2] Released antigens, which are short stretches of amino acids, are then presented by two different classes of major histocompatibility complex (MHC) molecules. MHC class 1 is expressed by all nucleated cells, whereas MHC class 2 molecules are constitutively expressed by APCs, such as dendritic cells and macrophages. Antigen presentation is a complex phenomenon essential for T-lymphocyte function.

T-Lymphocyte Activation, Localization, and Response

The interaction between the T-cell receptor complex and the MHC influences the immune response. The T-cell receptor complex consists of a highly variable CD4 or CD8 subunit that binds to MHC. MHC class 1 is recognized by CD8[+] T cells, whereas MHC class 2 is recognized by CD4[+] T cells. The T-cell receptor also consists of a CD3 molecule, which plays a role in relaying extracellular signaling to intracellular effector molecules. Successful immune activation requires two components. First, the variable CD4 or CD8 molecule must bind to an appropriately matched antigen. Second, this binding must occur in the presence of other costimulatory signals. Without sufficient costimulatory signals, antigen tolerance (or anergy) occurs.[3] The most important costimulatory signal in T cells is the binding of CD28 on lymphocytes to B7-1 (CD80) and B7-2 (CD86) on the APCs. Costimulation is tightly regulated by positively stimulating agonist molecules and negatively regulating immune checkpoint molecules, including cytotoxic T-lymphocyte-associated protein 4 (CTLA-4) and programmed cell death-1 (PD-1), which have become important targets for cancer immunotherapy agents.

Activation of T lymphocytes is followed by clonal expansion, wherein many copies of lymphocytes are created that share affinity with and specificity of the same antigen. A subset of these clonal lymphocytes become memory cells and a subset become effector cells. Effector lymphocytes are then trafficked through the vascular system to areas of tumor. This T-lymphocyte homing is mediated by various chemokine signals, including CX3CL1, CX3CL9, and CX3CL10. T lymphocytes must then exit through the vascular endothelium and infiltrate the tumor. Lastly, these activated and homed T lymphocytes must recognize antigens to in turn promote tumor cell killing.

Tumor Escape

Immunologic tumor escape is the phenomenon by which tumor cells escape immune surveillance.[4] Tumors have the ability to evade each step of the cancer immunity cycle. Tumor cells have the ability to generate immune tolerance that in turn decreases antigen release. Escape of T-lymphocyte activation can occur by several mechanisms. This includes manipulation of the cytokine microenvironment through increased production of anti-inflammatory cytokines, such as interleukin (IL)-10, which directly and indirectly suppress T lymphocytes.[5] Tumor cells can also upregulate the expression of checkpoint molecules to negatively regulate costimulation.[6] T-lymphocyte tumor infiltration is inhibited by increased tumor production of growth factors, such as vascular endothelial growth factor.[7] Tumor cells may also escape recognition through decreased MHC class 1 molecule expression, resulting in reduced antigen presentation.[8,9]

STRATEGIES FOR CANCER IMMUNOTHERAPY

Knowledge of the tumor immune response has led to several strategies to harness these processes and develop rational, immune-based tumor therapies. These strategies include cytokine therapies, checkpoint inhibition drugs, and antitumor vaccines (**Fig. 1**).

Cytokine-Based Therapy

Cytokines are glycoproteins produced by immune cells to generate a local and systemic response. Cytokines play a role in initiating, sustaining, and regulating immune responses by stimulating T-cell growth and natural killer cells. Importantly, they create a nonspecific immune response. Cytokine-based therapy was the first type of tumor immunotherapy developed for urologic malignancies. IL-2, the first cytokine found to have therapeutic benefit, was discovered in 1976 by Robert Gallo, MD, and Francis Ruscetti, PhD.[10] IL-2 achieves a durable response in a subset of patients with renal cell carcinoma and leads to improved survival when combined with cytoreductive nephrectomy in patients with metastatic

disease.[11] IL-2 has also shown efficacy in advanced melanoma.[12] Interferon alfa-2b, which promotes CD8[+] lymphocytes, and bacille Calmette-Guérin, which induces cancer cells to produce cytokines and present tumor antigens to lymphocytes, have shown efficacy in superficial urothelial carcinoma.[13]

Checkpoint Inhibition

Immune checkpoints are physiologic constraints on unrestrained cytotoxic T-effector function. The interaction between PD-1, a transmembrane protein expressed on T cells, and PD-1 ligand (PD-L1), expressed on normal cells and many tumor cells, is an important checkpoint for T lymphocytes.[14] The prevalence of PD-L2, the other known ligand of PD-1, and its relationship to response to anti-PD-1 therapy is unknown. The PD-1 inhibitors that target ligand (ie, anti-PD-L1) as opposed to receptor (anti-PD-1) interfere with ligand binding to PD-L2, but the clinical relevance of these interactions remains uncertain.[15,16]

The binding of PD-1 and PD-L1 acts as a physiologic brake on unrestrained T-lymphocyte function. Binding of PD-1 to tumor cell PD-LI leads to

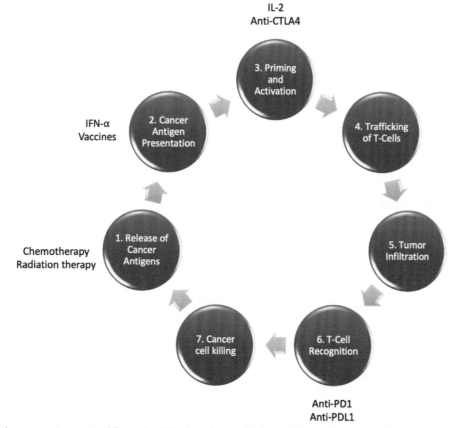

Fig. 1. The cancer-immunity life cycle. IFN, interferon. (*Adapted from* Chen, Daniel S., and Ira Mellman. "Oncology meets immunology: the cancer-immunity cycle." Immunity 39.1 (2013): 1-10.)

inhibition of tumor cell apoptosis and T-lymphocyte tolerance.[17] Checkpoint inhibitors are drugs that target these interactions. PD-1 inhibitors include pembrolizumab and nivolumab. PD-L1 inhibitors include atezolizumab, avelumab, and durvalumab. Currently, pembrolizumab is approved for microsatellite instability–high metastatic prostate cancer. Pembrolizumab and atezolizumab have been approved for use in metastatic urothelial cell carcinoma. Pembrolizumab has also been approved for use in bacille Calmette-Guérin–unresponsive, non–muscle invasive bladder cancer. Combination treatment with nivolumab and ipilimumab, pembrolizumab and axitinib, and avelumab and axitinib have been approved for advanced renal cell carcinoma.

CTLA-4 is a second transmembrane protein expressed on T lymphocytes and acts by competitively binding B7-1 (CD80) and B7-2 (CD86), located on APCs, to form a negative feedback loop on activated lymphocytes. The anti-CTLA-4 antibody ipilimumab was the first immune checkpoint inhibitor to be approved for metastatic cancer.[18]

Vaccines

Vaccines generate an adaptive immune response by relying on a combination of antigen presentation and accompanying immune adjuvants, which act to create the necessary immune microenvironment to stimulate immune cells. Vaccine antigens can be peptides, which are easier to prepare but limited in spectrum, or whole cell, which offers a broader range of antigens but are more labor intensive to generate. Viral-based cancer vaccines, such as ProstVac-VF, have also been developed for prostate cancer. Sipuleucel-T, a dendritic cell vaccine for advanced prostate cancer, is the only currently approved cancer vaccine. Dendritic cell vaccines are unique in that they rely on ex vivo manipulation. Dendritic cells are removed from the patient's body and isolated. The cells are subsequently primed to an antigen and these primed, antigen-presenting dendritic cells are reintroduced to the patient.

IMMUNOTHERAPY CONSIDERATIONS FOR PROSTATE CANCER

Although the basics of tumor immunobiology apply to all solid tumors, there are several important considerations specific to implementing immunotherapy for prostate cancer. The development of immunotherapy strategies for prostate cancer has differed slightly when compared with other solid tumors. For instance, therapeutic cancer vaccines have shown greater clinical activity in prostate cancer than in other tumor types. This is most notably because prostate cancer cells express several tumor-associated antigens. These cancer-specific antigens can be used to develop vaccines, which function by enhancing the immune recognition of these antigens to generate a targeted T-lymphocyte-mediated immune response. Several unique tumor-associated antigens are produced by prostate cells. Examples include prostatic acid phosphatase, which may regulate prostate cancer cell growth; prostate-specific antigen (PSA), which serves as a sensitive biomarker for low-volume disease and recurrence; and prostate-specific membrane antigen, a transmembrane protein that is induced to higher expression levels with androgen deprivation therapy (ADT).[19,20]

Despite the promise of vaccines in prostate cancer, results of treatment with other forms of immunotherapy, such as with checkpoint inhibitors, have been less robust compared with other malignancies.[21,22] Relative to other tumor types, prostate cancer cells have a low tumor mutational burden and a low expression of PD-L1.[23,24] Similarly, prostate cancer is a "cold" tumor with minimal T-cell infiltrates.[25] Furthermore, prostate cancer characteristically has absent or downregulated MHC class 1 expression, in primary and metastatic tumors, posing a challenge for immunotherapy agents, such as checkpoint inhibitors, which rely on MHC class 1–mediated antigen presentation.[26,27] These factors have been challenges for implementing newer forms of immunotherapy for prostate cancer.

In addition to differing responses to types of immunotherapy, there are important treatment-related and disease-related considerations that are specific to prostate cancer. For example, hormonal therapy, a cornerstone of prostate cancer treatment, has numerous implications related to immunotherapy. ADT has been shown to modulate the immune system by restoring thymic function and promoting T-cell proliferation.[28] In addition to these systemic effects, ADT leads to increased prostate immune infiltrates, increased cancer-targeted antigens, and decreased T-cell antigen tolerance. Together, these results suggest that hormonal therapy should augment the effect of immunotherapy.

In contrast, the predilection for prostate cancer to metastasize to bone proves to be a challenge in implementing immunotherapy. The bone microenvironment is oxygen poor and rich in lymphocyte regulatory cells and myeloid-derived suppressor cells, which act to dampen the immune response.[29] Furthermore, prostate cancer cells promote osteoblast- and osteoclast-mediated growth factor production. Many of these growth factors, such as transforming growth factor-β, suppress the immune response (**Table 1**).[30]

Several clinical trials have investigated the impact of immunotherapy on metastatic prostate cancer. In addition to advanced disease, there is growing rationale for and use of immunotherapy in localized disease. Importantly, unlike cytotoxic therapy, immunotherapy may not cause dramatic changes in tumor burden over a short period of time and relies on immunologic memory. Accordingly, starting immunotherapy earlier in the disease course may lead to much greater improvements in outcomes than starting later.[31] Vaccine-based therapies that have been studied include ProstVac-VF and Sipuleucel-T. Various checkpoint inhibitors, including ipilimumab, a humanized anti-CTLA-4 monoclonal antibody, and pembrolizumab, a PD-1 inhibitor, have also been studied (**Table 2**).

ProstVac-VF

ProstVac-VF is a viral-based recombinant vaccine that uses viral vectors containing transgenes for PSA and multiple proprietary T-cell costimulatory molecules (TRICOM) that act to bolster the local immune response.

Mechanisms

Primary vaccination is done using a vaccinia virus vector and subsequent booster doses are given using a fowlpox virus vector. The vaccinia virus produces a strong immune response with a single dose. However, if given in repeated doses, it is neutralized by the host immune response.[32] As such, subsequent doses are given using fowlpox, which although able to penetrate APCs, does not lead to production of high volumes of neutralizing antibodies by the host.[33]

ProstVac-VF in Advanced Prostate Cancer

Several clinical trials have evaluated the safety and efficacy of ProstVac-VF monotherapy. Initial phase I trials established the safety of vaccinia-based vaccines and subsequently of combined regimens of vaccinia virus priming with fowlpox virus boost.[34,35] In addition to establishing safety, these trials showed a tissue immune response and a PSA response. Several phase II trials of ProstVac-VF monotherapy for advanced prostate cancer again confirmed a PSA response and suggested an improvement in survival.[36,37]

Although a large phase III trial of 1200 chemotherapy-naive men with asymptomatic metastatic castration-resistant prostate cancer (mCRPC) showed no improvement in overall or progression-free survival between men randomized to ProstVac-VF or to placebo,[38] there is robust biologic and early clinical evidence to suggest that combining vaccine-based immunotherapy with traditional advanced prostate cancer therapies, including chemotherapy, androgen-targeted therapy, and bone radionucleotides, may improve outcomes. Docetaxel leads to tumor cell cytolysis, which in turn leads to an increase in tumor-associated antigens. Furthermore, preclinical data have suggested that docetaxel and other chemotherapeutic agents may have an immunostimulatory effect, by increasing cytokine production and increasing MHC class I expression.[39] A phase II study of docetaxel plus vaccine treatment showed that patients who received vaccine had an increase in antigen-specific T cells and a longer progression-free survival on docetaxel.[40] Larger studies of combination immunotherapy and chemotherapy are ongoing. In addition to chemotherapy, there is biologic probability that vaccine-based therapies may have increased efficacy with androgen-targeted therapies. Testosterone has an antiproliferative effect on T cells and ADT is known to enhance T-cell infiltration of the prostate.[41,42]

Studies combining vaccine-based treatments with newer androgen-targeted therapies, such as abiraterone or enzalutamide, are lacking. However, early results from a randomized phase II study of flutamide with or without vaccine in non-mCRPC have shown longer progression-free survival in the arm treated with vaccine compared with those treated with antiandrogen alone.[43] Along with androgens, other studies have looked at the impact of combining ProstVac-VF with bone-targeting therapies in men with bone mCRPC. Radiation treatment of tumors, even at low doses, is thought to increase tumor antigen generation and presentation. Sm-153 consists of radioactive samarium and a tetraphosphate chelator and acts by targeting low levels of radiation to metastatic lesions in bone. A phase II study of men with nonvisceral mCRPC showed longer progression-free survival (3.7 months vs 1.7 months; $P = .041$) and PSA response in men treated with Sm-153 combined with vaccine therapy compared with those treated with Sm-153 alone.[44]

ProstVac-VF in Localized Prostate Cancer

Phase I clinical trials have shown that of ProstVac-VF generates an inflammatory response in localized prostate cancer.[45] Studies of ProstVac-VF in early stage prostate cancer are ongoing. A

Table 1
Immunotherapies for prostate cancer

Drug Classes	Specific Agents	Mechanism	Applicability to Localized Prostate Cancer
Vaccine-Based Treatment			
Virus-based vaccine	PROSTVAC-VF[34]	Vaccinia and fowlpox virus genetically engineered to contain human PSA	Possible Ongoing phase II trial (NCT02326805) in patients with clinically localized prostate cancer on active surveillance. Primary outcome is tumor immune response.[46]
Dendritic cell vaccine	Sipuleucel-T[51]	Autologous dendritic cell vaccine to enhance T-cell response to prostatic acid phosphatase	Possible A current trial (NCT03686683) is examining the impact on active surveillance patients. Primary outcome is reduction in reclassification to a higher Gleason grade.[88]
Checkpoint Inhibitors			
PD-1 inhibitor	Pembrolizumab, nivolumab[60,61]	Monoclonal antibody against inhibitor molecule PD-1 expressed on T-cells	Unknown Pembrolizumab plus prostatic cryotherapy evaluated in men with low-volume hormone-sensitive metastatic prostate cancer. Results showed that 42% (5/12) of patients had a PSAs of <0.6 ng/mL at 1 y.[67]
PD-L1 inhibitor	Atezolizumab, avelumab, durvalumab[89]	Monoclonal antibody against inhibitor molecule PD-1 ligand expressed on tissue cells	Unknown
CTLA-4 inhibitor	Ipilimumab[56]	Monoclonal antibody against inhibitor molecule cytotoxic T-lymphocyte-associated protein 4	Unknown A phase I trial of the CTLA-4 inhibitor ipilimumab plus ADT in men with PSA only recurrent prostate cancer after local treatment showed improved PSA kinetics with the addition of immunotherapy.[64]

randomized phase II trial of ProstVac-VF in patients with clinically localized prostate cancer on active surveillance has completed accrual and follow-up.[46] Patients with low- or intermediate-risk prostate cancer (stage ≤T2a, grade group ≤2 [Gleason ≤3 + 4 = 7], ≤50% of the biopsy cores containing cancer, and PSA <20 ng/mL) were randomized (2:1) to 5 months of treatment with either vaccine or placebo. Prostate biopsy was performed following treatment. The primary outcome is tumor immune response as defined by tissue and serum biomarkers. Results from

this study are expected in 2021 (ClinicalTrials. gov NCT02326805).

There has also been interest in combining ProstVac-VF with radiation therapy for localized cancer. Radiation treatment can induce tumors to upregulate expression of MHC molecules and tumor-associated antigens, thereby making these cells more susceptible to a T-lymphocyte response.[47] Initial phase II studies of vaccine plus radiation therapy treatment showed an increase in PSA-specific T cells among patients treated with vaccine compared with control

Table 2
Selected clinical trials of immunotherapy for prostate cancer

Trial	Phase	Arms	N	Patient Population	Primary End Point	Median OS (mo); ORR[a]	Hazard Ratio (CI) vs Placebo
Kantoff et al,[53] 2010	3	Sipeulecel-T vs placebo	512	mCRPC	OS	25.8 vs 21.7	0.78 (0.61–0.98)
Kwon et al,[56] 2014	3	Radiotherapy with ipilimumab vs placebo	799	mCRPC progressed on docetaxel	OS	11.2 vs 10.0	0.85 (0.72–1.00)
Beer et al,[57] 2017	3	Ipilimumab vs placebo	602	Asymptomatic mCRPC without prior therapy	OS	28.7 vs 29.7	1.11 (0.88–1.39)
Hansen et al,[60] 2018, KEYNOTE-028	1b	Pembrolizumab	23	Metastatic prostate cancer failing prior therapy with PD-L1 expression in ≥1%	ORR	17.4%	n/a[a]
Antonarakis et al,[59] 2020, KEYNOTE-199	2	Pembrolizumab	258	mCRPC treated with docetaxel and >1 targeted endocrine therapy with PD-L1-positive (cohort 1) or PD-L1-negative (cohort 2) disease	ORR	5% (cohort 1) and 3% (cohort 2)	n/a[a]
Sharma et al,[58] 2019 CheckMate 650	2	Nivolumab + ipilimumab	78	Asymptomatic mCRPC who progressed after second-generation hormone therapy without prior chemotherapy (cohort 1) vs patients who progressed after taxane therapy (cohort 2)	ORR	26% (cohort 1) and 10% (cohort 2)	n/a[a]

Abbreviations: CI, confidence interval; mCRPC, metastatic castration-resistant prostate cancer; ORR, objective response rate; OS, overall survival.
[a] Patients enrolled in KEYNOTE-028, KEYNOTE-199, and CheckMate 650 were nonrandomized.

subjects.[48] However, studies with longer term follow-up have shown that the addition of vaccine does not seem to have a significant difference with regard to PSA control and that long-term immune response may be limited.[49]

SIPULEUCEL-T

Sipuleucel-T is an autologous dendritic cell vaccine that enhances the immune response to prostatic acid phosphatase antigen. It is the only currently approved vaccine-based therapy for advanced cancer. In the setting of CRPC, Sipuleucel-T has had a favorable safety profile and prolonged survival compared with placebo.

Mechanisms

To prepare the vaccine, peripheral blood mononuclear cells are isolated by leukapheresis.[50] These cells are exposed ex vivo to a prostatic acid phosphatase antigen fused to human granulocyte-macrophage colony–stimulating factor. Once cells are activated to the antigen, they are infused back into the patient. A total of three treatments are performed over a 6-week period.[51]

Sipuleucel-T in Advanced Prostate Cancer

Evidence for the efficacy of Sipuleucel-T in CRPC has come from three large randomized trials. Patients eligible for inclusion in these trials had radiologic evidence of asymptomatic or minimally symptomatic mCRPC and good performance status, defined as an Eastern Cooperative Oncology Group score of less than 1. A total of 225 men were evaluated in a pooled analysis of two separate trials. Results showed that when compared with placebo, treatment with Sipuleucel-T was associated with an improved, albeit statistically nonsignificant, progression-free survival (11.1 vs 9.7 months; $P = .11$). Overall survival, a secondary end point, was significantly longer in the Sipuleucel-T group compared with placebo (median, 23.2 vs 18.9 months; $P = .01$).[50,52] The phase III IMPACT trial evaluated overall survival as the primary end point.[53] A total of 512 patients were randomized in a 2:1 ratio to receive either Sipuleucel-T (341 patients) or placebo (171 patients). Among men receiving Sipuleucel-T, there was a relative reduction of 22% in the risk of death as compared with the placebo group (hazard ratio [HR], 0.78; $P = .03$). Median survival was improved by 4.1 months in the treatment group (25.8 months in the Sipuleucel-T group vs 21.7 months in the placebo group). Patients receiving vaccine had more frequent T-cell proliferation responses to prostatic acid phosphatase. Among patients receiving Sipuleucel-T, results from this study also showed that patients with an antibody response to vaccine antigens had a significantly longer survival.[53] In all three trials, Sipuleucel-T was generally well tolerated, with the most common adverse events being chills (53%), fatigue (41%), fever (31%), nausea (21%), and headache (7%).

Sipuleucel-T in Localized Prostate Cancer

The use of Sipuleucel-T in localized prostate cancer has garnered some interest. Tumor immune recruitment was analyzed in a study of 42 patients given a standard dose of Sipuleucel-T before radical prostatectomy. Results from this study showed a systemic and local tumor response to vaccine treatment. Patients given vaccine had higher peripheral levels of interferon-γ and increased T-cell proliferation. Immunohistochemistry results of tumor specimens showed an increase in cytotoxic and nonregulatory helper T cells.[54]

A current trial (NCT03686683) is examining the impact of Sipuleucel-T administered to active surveillance patients for newly diagnosed prostate cancer: the open label trial ProVent. This study is designed to accrue 450 participants with International Society of Urologic Pathology grade group 1 or 2 prostate cancer diagnosed via either systematic or MRI-targeted biopsy enrolled in active surveillance. The primary outcome of interest is the efficacy of Sipuleucel-T in reducing histopathologic reclassification to a higher Gleason grade within 36 months in prostate cancer subjects on active surveillance. This trial completed accrual ahead of schedule and is currently in follow-up.

CHECKPOINT INHIBITOR IMMUNOTHERAPY

Immune checkpoints act as negative feedbacks on T lymphocytes. CTLA-4, a molecule found on T lymphocytes, is an important inhibitory costimulatory signal that suppresses the T-cell response to antigen presentation when binding to B7 on APCs. PD-1 is a second inhibitory transmembrane protein expressed on T cells that acts by binding PD-L1, found on normal tissue cells. Checkpoint inhibitors act by blocking these signals to in turn stimulate the immune response.

Checkpoint Inhibitors in Advanced Prostate Cancer

Ipilimumab, a humanized anti-CTLA-4 monoclonal antibody, binds to the CTLA-4 receptor on T cells and augments the immune response by blocking the interaction of CTLA-4. Phase I/II trials have shown that ipilimumab is well tolerated alone and when combined with bone-targeted radiotherapy and may produce a PSA response.[55] However, two large phase III studies of ipilimumab have failed to show any improvement in overall survival over placebo. In both trials ipilimumab was given every 3 weeks for four cycles in men with CRPC. Among 799 patients with bone mCRPC who had received prior treatment with docetaxel, the combination of bone-directed radiotherapy plus immunotherapy showed no benefit in the primary outcome of overall survival when compared with placebo.[56] Median overall survival was 11.2 months (95% confidence interval [CI], 9.5–12.7) in men treated with ipilimumab and 10.0 months (95% CI, 8.3–11.0) with placebo (HR, 0.85; 95% CI, 0.72–1.00). Secondary analyses showed that median progression-free survival was improved with immunotherapy treatment compared with placebo (4.0 vs 3.1 months; HR, 0.70; 95% CI, 0.61–0.82). Also, a larger portion of patients treated with ipilimumab (13.1%; 95% CI, 9.5–17.5) had a greater than 50% PSA response when compared with placebo (5.2%; 95% CI, 3.0–8.4). A second trial, of 600 men with no prior nonhormonal treatment of asymptomatic or minimally symptomatic nonvisceral mCRPC, again compared therapy with ipilimumab versus placebo.[57] Results were similar, and no difference was seen in the primary outcome of overall survival. Median overall survival was 28.7 months (95% CI, 24.5–32.5 months) in the ipilimumab arm versus 29.7 months (95% CI, 26.1–34.2 months) in the placebo arm (HR, 1.11; 95.87% CI, 0.88–1.39). However, median progression-free survival was longer in the ipilimumab arm (5.6 vs 3.8 months; HR, 0.67; 95.87% CI, 0.55–0.81). PSA response also seemed to be higher in the treatment arm (23%; 95% CI, 19%–27%) than with placebo (8%; 95% CI, 5%–13%). Together these studies showed that immunotherapy for advanced prostate cancer has an acceptable and well-tolerated toxicity profile. Moreover, these trials have shown that despite inducing some measurable antitumor activity, via progression-free survival and PSA response, treatment with ipilimumab does not extend overall survival in unselected populations of patients with mCRPC. With the limited clinical benefit of checkpoint inhibitor monotherapy, ongoing trials are attempting to evaluate the efficacy of combination immunotherapy. The CheckMate 650 trial is aiming to evaluate the efficacy of nivolumab plus ipilimumab in men with mCRPC in two cohorts, those who have progressed after second-generation hormone therapy and have not received chemotherapy and those who have progressed after

taxane-based chemotherapy.[58] Interim results have shown objective response rates of 26% in chemotherapy-naive patients and 10% in those failing prior taxane therapy. Furthermore, objective response rates in both cohorts were higher among patients with PD-L1 expression greater than 1%, DNA damage repair or homologous recombination mutations, or higher tumor mutational burden.

The PD-1 inhibitor pembrolizumab has been studied in CRPC. KEYNOTE-199, a phase II trial of men with mCRPC who failed prior chemotherapy, enrolled 258 men.[59] Patients were stratified into three different cohorts based on PD-L1 overexpression and location of metastatic disease. A total of 133 men had PD-L1-positive disease, 66 had PD-L1-negative disease, and 59 had bone-predominant disease. Among men with PD-L1 overexpression, there was a 5% objective response and a complete response in two patients. Among patients with bone-predominant disease, the disease control rate was 22%. Results from the smaller KEYNOTE-028 also suggested that pembrolizumab can result in durable responses for individuals with CRPC and PD-L1 overexpression.[60] Data from other cancers have suggested that in addition to PD-L1 expression, tumors with DNA mismatch repair mechanism (dMMR) mutations may derive benefit from treatment with pembrolizumab.[61] Tumors with dMMR mutations seem to have higher rates of mutations and a resultant higher rate of tumor-associated antigens. A hallmark of dMMR is the presence of high levels of microsatellite instability.[61] Based on data from other tumors, pembrolizumab is currently approved for treatment of a variety of advanced solid tumors, including prostate cancers, that have dMMR mutations or microsatellite instability, specifically in men who have progressed following prior treatment and exhausted alternative treatment options. However, results from other studies have suggested that dMMR mutations and microsatellite instability are rare in advanced prostate cancer, occurring as infrequently as 1% to 2%, limiting the widespread use of PD-L1 inhibitors in advanced prostate cancer.[62,63]

Checkpoint Inhibitors in Oligometastatic Prostate Cancer

As a treatment that relies on generating an immunogenic response with treatment memory, there is biologic rationale for starting checkpoint inhibitor therapy earlier in the disease course. A phase I trial of the CTLA-4 inhibitor ipilimumab plus ADT in men with PSA only recurrent prostate cancer after local treatment showed improved PSA kinetics with the addition of immunotherapy.[64] Some research has posited that adding local therapy to systemic immunotherapy may be more effective than immunotherapy given alone. Localized cell death leads to increased immune presentation that may augment a systemic response, a phenomenon known as the abscopal effect.[65] Preclinical models have suggested that, among forms of local treatment, cryotherapy may produce the most robust immune response.[66] With this evidence in mind, a recent trial evaluated the potential benefit of combining pembrolizumab plus prostatic cryotherapy among men with low volume (≤5 metastases) hormone-sensitive metastatic prostate cancer.[67] Treatment was well tolerated with minimal complications. Results from this study showed that 42% (5/12) of patients had PSAs of less than 0.6 ng/mL at 1 year.

Checkpoint Inhibitors in Localized Prostate Cancer

Treatment with checkpoint inhibitors before surgery for prostate cancer has been investigated. A total of 20 patients with localized, high-risk prostate cancer were treated with ADT and two doses of ipilimumab before radical prostatectomy.[68] Tumor specimens were analyzed to better understand prostate tumor immune response. The authors discovered potential compensatory immune inhibitory pathways that may arise in the setting of immune checkpoint inhibition. After treatment with checkpoint inhibitor therapy, tumors had significantly higher levels of PD-1 and PD-L1 expression and increased expression of VISTA, a second inhibitor molecule known to suppress T-lymphocyte response.[69] The results from this study have helped elucidate possible mechanisms of prostate cancer's relative resistance to immune monotherapy.

FUTURE DIRECTIONS
Combination Therapies

Despite the disappointing results of checkpoint inhibitor monotherapy in advanced prostate cancer, there is increasing evidence that combining checkpoint inhibitors with other forms of systemic therapy may enhance their efficacy. Tyrosine kinase inhibitors may perform synergistically with checkpoint inhibitors by allowing for increased tumor perfusion and lymphocyte infiltration.[70] A recent phase 1b study (COSMIC-021) investigated the objective response rate of patients with mCRPC treated with the tyrosine kinase inhibitor cabozantinib combined with the PD-L1 inhibitor atezolizumab. Results showed an objective response rate of 32%, with 4.5% having a complete response and 27% having a partial response.[71] Other trials using a similar approach include an ongoing phase I study investigating tremelimumab (anti-CTLA-4) plus durvalumab (anti-PD-L1) in patients with chemotherapy-naive mCRPC (NCT03204812) and the IMPACT study (NCT03570619) of nivolumab plus ipilimumab in populations with mutations in CDK12. CDK12 mutations, which are present in approximately 5% of mCRPC tumors, confer a distinct phenotype of prostate cancer that is thought to be more immunogenic.[72]

Another approach would be to combine different treatment modalities to potentiate immunotherapies for localized disease. Pairing an established prostate ablation therapy, such as cryoablation, with a checkpoint inhibitor or cancer vaccine holds conceptual promise. Cryoablation lyses tumor cells and provokes a systemic immune response. Treating a prostate tumor with cryoablation would potentially prime it for subsequent immunotherapy by turning a "cold" prostate cancer "hot" and thus rendering it more susceptible to a cancer vaccine or checkpoint inhibitor.[73,74]

T-Cell Engaging Therapies

A promising technology in development is the use genetic engineering for immunotherapy. These treatments include chimeric lymphocytes and bispecific antibodies. Chimeric antigen receptor (CAR) T lymphocytes are genetically engineered cells designed to produce an artificial T-lymphocyte receptor for use in immunotherapy. An ongoing phase I trial is investigating the safety of CAR T lymphocytes directed at prostate-specific membrane antigen. Initial cohorts have completed therapy with no reports of dose-limiting toxicity.[75] A phase I study of CAR-T (NCT04249947) began actively recruiting in January 2020. Bispecific antibodies are genetically engineered antibody proteins that are designed to bind to two different types of antigens. By binding tumor antigens in one arm and T-lymphocyte antigens in the second arm, tumor cells are more effectively cross-linked to effector immune cells.[76] Bispecific antibodies that target the tumor antigen prostate-specific membrane antigen and the T-lymphocyte antigen CD3 have recently been developed for prostate cancer, with early results indicating promising tolerability.[77] A phase I trial (NCT03577028) investigating the efficacy of the bispecific antibody HPN424 is currently accruing patients with CRPC.

Predictors of Immune Response

With immunotherapy becoming more widely used in advanced cancer treatment, there has been increased effort in understanding potential predictors of response to treatment. Several predictors of immune response have been studied, including PD-L1 expression via immunohistochemistry, tumor mutational burden, gene expression profiling, and multiplex immunohistochemistry/immunofluorescence. These assays have been used to assess pretreatment tumor tissue to predict response to checkpoint inhibitor treatment.[78] Results among men with CRPC suggest that PD-L1 overexpression may predict response to agents that target this pathway. However, many prostate tumors lack PD-L1 expression.[24] Results suggest that men with intraductal tumors, high-grade (grade group 5) tumors, and tumors that are resistant to enzalutamide may have greater levels of PD-L1 expression.[79–81] Other authors have suggested that PD-L2 may be an alternative marker in prostate tumors to predict immunotherapy response.[22] Tumor mutational burden is a well-established marker of response to PD-1 inhibition.[82] However, relative to other solid tumors, prostate cancers tend to have a lower mutational burden. The advent of large-scale and rapid-throughput gene-expression profiling of tumors has led to development of several gene signatures that have shown to predict response to immunotherapy.[83]

Specifically, biallelic inactivation of CDK12 is a promising marker for immunogenic prostate cancer. CDK12 is a cyclin-dependent kinase that controls genetic stability by regulating DNA repair genes. CDK12 mutation is associated with increased genomic instability and leads to increased gene fusion events and neoantigen creation. Tumors with CDK12 mutations also have increased lymphocyte infiltration.[84] Several gene profiles have been developed in metastatic melanoma and non–small cell lung cancer.[85] Many of these genes are immune related and involve chemokine pathways. However, these have yet to be developed or validated for prostate cancer. The immune characteristic of the tumor microenvironment provides an additional way to predict treatment response. With this aim in mind, multiplex immunohistochemistry/immunofluorescence is a novel method of staining immune cells and tumors cells. This technique provides objective, quantitative data describing the immune subset and location within the tumor microenvironment. These data are used to better classify tumors as being T-lymphocyte inflamed versus immune excluded.[86]

In addition to tumor specific predictors of response, increasing evidence suggests that response to immunotherapy involves a complex interplay between somatic inheritance and tumor-related mutations. MHC molecules are highly genetically variable. Recent results have shown that inherited MHC class I genotype plays a role in restricting the ability of T lymphocytes to present certain tumor antigens.[87] As such, future efforts to predict response to immunotherapy may rely on combining patient-specific and tumor-specific data to optimize candidates for this type of therapy.

FUNDING

Dr. Mckay: NCI P30CA023100-34 Prostate Cancer Foundation Young Investigator Award.

SUMMARY

Compared with other solid tumors, prostate cancer poses challenges for immunotherapy. Whereas the vaccine-based treatment Sipuleucel-T has been introduced in the clinic, other immunotherapy agents, including checkpoint inhibitors, have shown limited efficacy in prostate cancer. Ongoing trials of combination therapy may enhance the efficacy of checkpoint inhibitors for advanced prostate cancer. Biomarkers for immunotherapy response, including mutations in CDK12, also show promise. New treatments, including chimeric T lymphocytes and bispecific antibodies, provide future opportunities to enhance the immune response to prostate tumors.

REFERENCES

1. Hennecke J, Wiley DC. T cell receptor-MHC interactions up close. Cell 2001;104(1):1–4.
2. Boon T, Cerottini JC, Van den Eynde B, et al. Tumor antigens recognized by T lymphocytes. Annu Rev Immunol 1994;12:337–65.
3. Wherry EJ. T cell exhaustion. Nat Immunol 2011; 12(6):492–9.
4. Gajewski TF, Woo S-R, Zha Y, et al. Cancer immunotherapy strategies based on overcoming barriers within the tumor microenvironment. Curr Opin Immunol 2013;25(2):268–76.
5. Vinay DS, Ryan EP, Pawelec G, et al. Immune evasion in cancer: mechanistic basis and therapeutic strategies. Semin Cancer Biol 2015;35(Suppl): S185–98.
6. Tumeh PC, Harview CL, Yearley JH, et al. PD-1 blockade induces responses by inhibiting adaptive immune resistance. Nature 2014;515(7528):568–71.
7. Franciszkiewicz K, Le Floc'h A, Boutet M, et al. CD103 or LFA-1 engagement at the immune synapse between cytotoxic T cells and tumor cells promotes maturation and regulates T-cell effector functions. Cancer Res 2013;73(2):617–28.

8. Zaretsky JM, Garcia-Diaz A, Shin DS, et al. Mutations associated with acquired resistance to PD-1 blockade in melanoma. N Engl J Med 2016;375(9): 819–29.

9. Rooney MS, Shukla SA, Wu CJ, et al. Molecular and genetic properties of tumors associated with local immune cytolytic activity. Cell 2015;160(1–2):48–61.

10. Rosenberg SA, Mulé JJ, Spiess PJ, et al. Regression of established pulmonary metastases and subcutaneous tumor mediated by the systemic administration of high-dose recombinant interleukin 2. J Exp Med 1985;161(5):1169–88.

11. Belldegrun AS, Klatte T, Shuch B, et al. Cancer-specific survival outcomes among patients treated during the cytokine era of kidney cancer (1989-2005): a benchmark for emerging targeted cancer therapies. Cancer 2008;113(9):2457–63.

12. Rosenberg SA, Yang JC, Topalian SL, et al. Treatment of 283 consecutive patients with metastatic melanoma or renal cell cancer using high-dose bolus interleukin 2. JAMA 1994;271(12):907–13.

13. Redelman-Sidi G, Glickman MS, Bochner BH. The mechanism of action of BCG therapy for bladder cancer: a current perspective. Nat Rev Urol 2014; 11(3):153–62.

14. Spranger S, Spaapen RM, Zha Y, et al. Up-regulation of PD-L1, IDO, and T(regs) in the melanoma tumor microenvironment is driven by CD8(+) T cells. Sci Transl Med 2013;5(200):200ra116.

15. Yearley JH, Gibson C, Yu N, et al. PD-L2 expression in human tumors: relevance to anti-PD-1 therapy in cancer. Clin Cancer Res 2017;23(12):3158–67.

16. Yang H, Zhou X, Sun L, et al. Correlation between PD-L2 expression and clinical outcome in solid cancer patients: a meta-analysis. Front Oncol 2019;9:47.

17. Francisco LM, Salinas VH, Brown KE, et al. PD-L1 regulates the development, maintenance, and function of induced regulatory T cells. J Exp Med 2009; 206(13):3015–29.

18. Schadendorf D, Hodi FS, Robert C, et al. Pooled analysis of long-term survival data from phase II and phase III trials of ipilimumab in unresectable or metastatic melanoma. J Clin Oncol 2015;33(17): 1889–94.

19. Kong HY, Byun J. Emerging roles of human prostatic acid phosphatase. Biomol Ther (Seoul) 2013;21(1):10–20.

20. Wright GL, Grob BM, Haley C, et al. Upregulation of prostate-specific membrane antigen after androgen-deprivation therapy. Urology 1996;48(2):326–34.

21. Madan RA, Gulley JL. Finding an immunologic beachhead in the prostate cancer microenvironment. J Natl Cancer Inst 2019;111(3):219–20.

22. Zhao SG, Lehrer J, Chang SL, et al. The immune landscape of prostate cancer and nomination of PD-L2 as a potential therapeutic target. J Natl Cancer Inst 2019;111(3):301–10.

23. Cancer Genome Atlas Research Network. The molecular taxonomy of primary prostate cancer. Cell 2015;163(4):1011–25.

24. Martin AM, Nirschl TR, Nirschl CJ, et al. Paucity of PD-L1 expression in prostate cancer: innate and adaptive immune resistance. Prostate Cancer Prostatic Dis 2015;18(4):325–32.

25. Vitkin N, Nersesian S, Siemens DR, et al. The tumor immune contexture of prostate cancer. Front Immunol 2019;10:603.

26. Blades RA, Keating PJ, McWilliam LJ, et al. Loss of HLA class I expression in prostate cancer: implications for immunotherapy. Urology 1995;46(5):681–6 [discussion: 686–7].

27. Sanda MG, Restifo NP, Walsh JC, et al. Molecular characterization of defective antigen processing in human prostate cancer. J Natl Cancer Inst 1995; 87(4):280–5.

28. Brelińska R. Thymic epithelial cells in age-dependent involution. Microsc Res Tech 2003; 62(6):488–500.

29. Ahern E, Harjunpää H, Barkauskas D, et al. Co-administration of RANKL and CTLA4 antibodies enhances lymphocyte-mediated antitumor immunity in mice. Clin Cancer Res 2017;23(19):5789–801.

30. Thomas DA, Massagué J. TGF-beta directly targets cytotoxic T cell functions during tumor evasion of immune surveillance. Cancer Cell 2005;8(5):369–80.

31. Gulley JL, Madan RA, Schlom J. Impact of tumour volume on the potential efficacy of therapeutic vaccines. Curr Oncol 2011;18(3):e150–7.

32. Gulley J, Chen AP, Dahut W, et al. Phase I study of a vaccine using recombinant vaccinia virus expressing PSA (rV-PSA) in patients with metastatic androgen-independent prostate cancer. Prostate 2002;53(2):109–17.

33. Hodge JW, McLaughlin JP, Kantor JA, et al. Diversified prime and boost protocols using recombinant vaccinia virus and recombinant non-replicating avian pox virus to enhance T-cell immunity and antitumor responses. Vaccine 1997;15(6–7):759–68.

34. Eder JP, Kantoff PW, Roper K, et al. A phase I trial of a recombinant vaccinia virus expressing prostate-specific antigen in advanced prostate cancer. Clin Cancer Res 2000;6(5):1632–8. Available at: http://www.ncbi.nlm.nih.gov/pubmed/10815880.

35. Arlen PM, Skarupa L, Pazdur M, et al. Clinical safety of a viral vector based prostate cancer vaccine strategy. J Urol 2007;178(4 Pt 1):1515–20.

36. Kaufman HL, Wang W, Manola J, et al. Phase II randomized study of vaccine treatment of advanced prostate cancer (E7897): a trial of the Eastern Cooperative Oncology Group. J Clin Oncol 2004;22(11): 2122–32.

37. Kantoff PW, Schuetz TJ, Blumenstein BA, et al. Overall survival analysis of a phase II randomized controlled trial of a Poxviral-based PSA-targeted

immunotherapy in metastatic castration-resistant prostate cancer. J Clin Oncol 2010;28(7):1099–105.

38. Gulley JL, Borre M, Vogelzang NJ, et al. Phase III trial of PROSTVAC in asymptomatic or minimally symptomatic metastatic castration-resistant prostate cancer. J Clin Oncol 2019;37(13):1051–61.

39. Chan OTM, Yang LX. The immunological effects of taxanes. Cancer Immunol Immunother 2000;49(4–5):181–5.

40. Arlen PM, Gulley JL, Parker C, et al. A randomized phase II study of concurrent docetaxel plus vaccine versus vaccine alone in metastatic androgen-independent prostate cancer. Clin Cancer Res 2006;12(4):1260–9.

41. Sutherland JS, Goldberg GL, Hammett MV, et al. Activation of thymic regeneration in mice and humans following androgen blockade. J Immunol 2005;175(4):2741–53.

42. Drake CG, Doody ADH, Mihalyo MA, et al. Androgen ablation mitigates tolerance to a prostate/prostate cancer-restricted antigen. Cancer Cell 2005;7(3):239–49.

43. Bilusic A-M, Gulley A-JL, Heery A-C, et al. A randomized phase II study of flutamide with or without PSA-TRICOM in nonmetastatic castration-resistant prostate cancer (CRPC). J Clin Oncol 2011;29:163.

44. Heery CR, Madan RA, Stein MN, et al. Samarium-153-EDTMP (Quadramet) with or without vaccine in metastatic castration-resistant prostate cancer: a randomized phase 2 trial. Oncotarget 2016;7(42):69014–23.

45. Merino MJ, Pinto PA, Moreno V, et al. Morphological changes induced by intraprostatic PSA-based vaccine in prostate cancer biopsies (phase I clinical trial). Hum Pathol 2018;78:72–8.

46. Parsons JK, Pinto PA, Pavlovich CP, et al. A randomized, double-blind, phase II Trial of PSA-TRICOM (PROSTVAC) in patients with localized prostate cancer: the immunotherapy to prevent progression on active surveillance study. Eur Urol Focus 2018;4(5):636–8.

47. Sheard MA, Vojtesek B, Janakova L, et al. Up-regulation of Fas (CD95) in human p53wild-type cancer cells treated with ionizing radiation. Int J Cancer 1997;73(5):757–62.

48. Gulley JL, Arlen PM, Bastian A, et al. Combining a recombinant cancer vaccine with standard definitive radiotherapy in patients with localized prostate cancer. Clin Cancer Res 2005;11(9):3353–62.

49. Kamrava M, Kesarwala AH, Madan RA, et al. Long-term follow-up of prostate cancer patients treated with vaccine and definitive radiation therapy. Prostate Cancer Prostatic Dis 2012;15(3):289–95.

50. Higano CS, Schellhammer PF, Small EJ, et al. Integrated data from 2 randomized, double-blind, placebo-controlled, phase 3 trials of active cellular immunotherapy with sipuleucel-T in advanced prostate cancer. Cancer 2009;115(16):3670–9.

51. Tanimoto T, Hori A, Kami M. Sipuleucel-T immunotherapy for castration-resistant prostate cancer. N Engl J Med 2010;363(20):1966 [author reply: 1967–8].

52. Small EJ, Schellhammer PF, Higano CS, et al. Placebo-controlled phase III trial of immunologic therapy with sipuleucel-T (APC8015) in patients with metastatic, asymptomatic hormone refractory prostate cancer. J Clin Oncol 2006;24(19):3089–94.

53. Kantoff PW, Higano CS, Shore ND, et al. Sipuleucel-T immunotherapy for castration-resistant prostate cancer. N Engl J Med 2010;363(5):411–22.

54. Fong L, Carroll P, Weinberg V, et al. Activated lymphocyte recruitment into the tumor microenvironment following preoperative sipuleucel-T for localized prostate cancer. J Natl Cancer Inst 2014;106(11). https://doi.org/10.1093/jnci/dju268.

55. Slovin SF, Higano CS, Hamid O, et al. Ipilimumab alone or in combination with radiotherapy in metastatic castration-resistant prostate cancer: results from an open-label, multicenter phase I/II study. Ann Oncol 2013;24(7):1813–21.

56. Kwon ED, Drake CG, Scher HI, et al. Ipilimumab versus placebo after radiotherapy in patients with metastatic castration-resistant prostate cancer that had progressed after docetaxel chemotherapy (CA184-043): a multicentre, randomised, double-blind, phase 3 trial. Lancet Oncol 2014;15(7):700–12.

57. Beer TM, Kwon ED, Drake CG, et al. Randomized, double-blind, phase III trial of ipilimumab versus placebo in asymptomatic or minimally symptomatic patients with metastatic chemotherapy-naive castration-resistant prostate cancer. J Clin Oncol 2017;35(1):40–7.

58. Sharma P, Pachynski RK, Narayan V, et al. Initial results from a phase II study of nivolumab (NIVO) plus ipilimumab (IPI) for the treatment of metastatic castration-resistant prostate cancer (mCRPC; CheckMate 650). J Clin Oncol 2019;37(7_suppl):142.

59. Antonarakis ES, Piulats JM, Gross-Goupil M, et al. Pembrolizumab for treatment-refractory metastatic castration-resistant prostate cancer: multicohort, open-label phase II KEYNOTE-199 Study. J Clin Oncol 2020;JCO1901638. https://doi.org/10.1200/JCO.19.01638.

60. Hansen AR, Massard C, Ott PA, et al. Pembrolizumab for advanced prostate adenocarcinoma: findings of the KEYNOTE-028 study. Ann Oncol 2018;29(8):1807–13.

61. Le DT, Uram JN, Wang H, et al. PD-1 blockade in tumors with mismatch-repair deficiency. N Engl J Med 2015;372(26):2509–20.

62. Middha S, Zhang L, Nafa K, et al. Reliable pan-cancer microsatellite instability assessment by using targeted next-generation sequencing data. JCO Precis Oncol 2017;2017. https://doi.org/10.1200/PO.17.00084.

63. Abida W, Cheng ML, Armenia J, et al. Analysis of the prevalence of microsatellite instability in prostate cancer and response to immune checkpoint blockade. JAMA Oncol 2019;5(4):471–8.

64. Autio KA, Eastham JA, Danila DC, et al. A phase II study combining ipilimumab and degarelix with or without radical prostatectomy (RP) in men with newly diagnosed metastatic noncastration prostate cancer (mNCPC) or biochemically recurrent (BR) NCPC. J Clin Oncol 2017;35(6_suppl):203.

65. Abdo J, Cornell DL, Mittal SK, et al. Immunotherapy plus cryotherapy: potential augmented abscopal effect for advanced cancers. Front Oncol 2018;8:85.

66. Benzon B, Glavaris SA, Simons BW, et al. Combining immune check-point blockade and cryoablation in an immunocompetent hormone sensitive murine model of prostate cancer. Prostate Cancer Prostatic Dis 2018;21(1):126–36.

67. Ross AE, Hurley PJ, Tran PT, et al. A pilot trial of pembrolizumab plus prostatic cryotherapy for men with newly diagnosed oligometastatic hormone-sensitive prostate cancer. Prostate Cancer Prostatic Dis 2019. https://doi.org/10.1038/s41391-019-0176-8.

68. Gao J, Ward JF, Pettaway CA, et al. VISTA is an inhibitory immune checkpoint that is increased after ipilimumab therapy in patients with prostate cancer. Nat Med 2017;23(5):551–5.

69. Lines JL, Sempere LF, Broughton T, et al. VISTA is a novel broad-spectrum negative checkpoint regulator for cancer immunotherapy. Cancer Immunol Res 2014;2(6):510–7.

70. Kwilas AR, Ardiani A, Donahue RN, et al. Dual effects of a targeted small-molecule inhibitor (cabozantinib) on immune-mediated killing of tumor cells and immune tumor microenvironment permissiveness when combined with a cancer vaccine. J Transl Med 2014;12:294.

71. Agarwal N, Loriot Y, McGregor BA, et al. . Cabozantinib (C) in combination with atezolizumab (A) in patients (pts) with metastatic castration-resistant prostate cancer (mCRPC): results of Cohort 6 of the COSMIC-021 Study. J Clin Oncol 2020;38(6_supp):139.

72. Robinson D, Van Allen EM, Wu Y-M, et al. Integrative clinical genomics of advanced prostate cancer. Cell 2015;162(2):454.

73. Yakkala C, Chiang CL-L, Kandalaft L, et al. Cryoablation and immunotherapy: an enthralling synergy to confront the tumors. Front Immunol 2019;10:2283.

74. Schlom J, Gulley JL. Vaccines as an integral component of cancer immunotherapy. JAMA 2018;320(21):2195–6.

75. Narayan V, Gladney W, Plesa G, et al. A phase I clinical trial of PSMA-directed/TGFβ-insensitive CAR-T cells in metastatic castration-resistant prostate cancer. J Clin Oncol 2019;37(7_suppl):TPS347.

76. Sedykh SE, Prinz V, Buneva VN, et al. Bispecific antibodies: design, therapy, perspectives. Drug Des Devel Ther 2018;12:195–208.

77. Clarke S, Dang K, Li Y, et al. A novel CD3xPSMA bispecific antibody for efficient T cell mediated killing of prostate tumor cells with minimal cytokine release. J Clin Oncol 2019;37(7_suppl):324.

78. Lu S, Stein JE, Rimm DL, et al. Comparison of biomarker modalities for predicting response to PD-1/PD-L1 checkpoint blockade: a systematic review and meta-analysis. JAMA Oncol 2019. https://doi.org/10.1001/jamaoncol.2019.1549.

79. Bishop JL, Sio A, Angeles A, et al. PD-L1 is highly expressed in enzalutamide resistant prostate cancer. Oncotarget 2015;6(1):234–42.

80. Antonarakis ES, Shaukat F, Isaacsson Velho P, et al. Clinical features and therapeutic outcomes in men with advanced prostate cancer and DNA mismatch repair gene mutations. Eur Urol 2019;75(3):378–82.

81. Schweizer MT, Antonarakis ES, Bismar TA, et al. Genomic characterization of prostatic ductal adenocarcinoma identifies a high prevalence of DNA repair gene mutations. JCO Precis Oncol 2019;3. https://doi.org/10.1200/PO.18.00327.

82. Mutation burden predicts anti-PD-1 response. Cancer Discov 2018;8(3):258.

83. Jamieson NB, Maker AV. Gene-expression profiling to predict responsiveness to immunotherapy. Cancer Gene Ther 2017;24(3):134–40.

84. Wu Y-M, Cieślik M, Lonigro RJ, et al. Inactivation of CDK12 delineates a distinct immunogenic class of advanced prostate cancer. Cell 2018;173(7):1770–82.e14.

85. Ulloa-Montoya F, Louahed J, Dizier B, et al. Predictive gene signature in MAGE-A3 antigen-specific cancer immunotherapy. J Clin Oncol 2013;31(19):2388–95.

86. Hofman P, Badoual C, Henderson F, et al. Multiplexed immunohistochemistry for molecular and immune profiling in lung cancer-just about ready for prime-time? Cancers (Basel) 2019;11(3). https://doi.org/10.3390/cancers11030283.

87. Marty R, Kaabinejadian S, Rossell D, et al. MHC-I genotype restricts the oncogenic mutational landscape. Cell 2017;171(6):1272–83.e15.

88. Ross A, Armstrong AJ, Pieczonka CM, et al. A comparison of sipuleucel-T (sip-T) product parameters from two phase III studies: PROVENT in active surveillance prostate cancer and IMPACT in metastatic castrate-resistant prostate cancer (mCRPC). ASCO.:321.

89. Hodi FS, Ballinger M, Lyons B, et al. Immune-modified response evaluation criteria in solid tumors (imRECIST): refining guidelines to assess the clinical benefit of cancer immunotherapy. J Clin Oncol 2018;36(9):850–8.

The Potential Role for Immunotherapy in Biochemically Recurrent Prostate Cancer

Marijo Bilusic, MD[a], David J. Einstein, MD[b], Fatima H. Karzai, MD[a],
William L. Dahut, MD[a], James L. Gulley, MD[a], Jeanny B. Aragon-Ching, MD[c],
Ravi A. Madan, MD[a],*

KEYWORDS

• Systemic therapy • Immunotherapy-based treatment • Prostate cancer • Biochemically recurrent

KEY POINTS

- Currently, there is no clear standard of care for patients with biochemically recurrent prostate cancer and no systemic therapy has been shown to improve survival.
- Immunotherapy-based treatments are potentially attractive options relative to androgen deprivation therapy due to the generally more favorable side-effect profile.
- Biochemically recurrent prostate cancer patients have a low tumor burden and likely lymph node–based disease, which may make them more likely to respond to immunotherapy.
- As modern immunotherapeutic strategies converge with emerging imaging platforms, immunotherapy may find more opportunities for clinical success in biochemically recurrent prostate cancer than in more advanced disease states.

INTRODUCTION

Approximately 191,930 men will be diagnosed and 33,330 will die from prostate cancer in the United States in 2020.[1] Although the majority of patients can be cured with definitive local therapies, 20% to 40% of patients undergoing radical prostatectomy (RP) and 30% to 50% of those undergoing radiation therapy (RT) at some time point will experience treatment failure, known as biochemical recurrence (BCR) or nonmetastatic castration–sensitive prostate cancer.[2] This common disease state, with more than 25,000 new cases annually, is defined by a rising prostate-specific antigen (PSA) in the absence of visible metastases on conventional imaging (computed tomography [CT] or and technetium Tc 99m [Tc99] bone scan).[3,4] The PSA threshold is dependent on the type of local

therapy. PSA value greater than 0.2 ng/mL, measured between 6 weeks and 13 weeks after RP, followed by a repeated test confirming a persistent PSA greater than 0.2 ng/mL, is consistent with BCR.[5] On the other hand, BCR after RT is defined as a PSA rise of 2 ng/mL or more above the nadir, with or without androgen deprivation therapy (ADT) (Phoenix definition).[6] The Phoenix definition frequently has been used in clinical practice and has shown improved accuracy over the American Society for Radiation Oncology definition of BCR (defined as 3 consecutive PSA rises after a nadir) in predicting patient outcomes.[7]

In this asymptomatic phase, in a generally healthy population, the most effective management is still uncertain because no intervention has been shown to prolong survival. Consequently, there is no consensus on when to start

[a] Genitourinary Malignancies Branch, Center for Cancer Research, National Cancer Institute, 10 Center Drive, 13n240b, Bethesda, MD 20892, USA; [b] Division of Medical Oncology, Beth Israel Deaconess Medical Center, Boston, MA, USA; [c] GU Medical Oncology, Inova Schar Cancer Institute, Fairfax, VA, USA
* Corresponding author.
E-mail address: madanr@mail.nih.gov

Urol Clin N Am 47 (2020) 457–467
https://doi.org/10.1016/j.ucl.2020.07.004
0094-0143/20/Published by Elsevier Inc.

treatment. BCR is a heterogeneous disease with a variable clinical course: some patients have an indolent course for years and may never die from prostate cancer; others may have a rapid progression to metastatic disease with increased risk of mortality from prostate cancer. In a study evaluating BCR after RP, the median time from BCR to clinical progression was noted to be 8 years and from development of metastasis to prostate cancer–specific mortality (PCSM) was 5 years, indicating that median overall survival (OS) from the diagnosis of BCR was approximately 13 years.[8] Based on retrospective studies, BCR patients do have shorter survival (88% 10-year OS rate compared with the 93% 10-year OS rate in men without BCR).[9] This emphasizes the importance of a personalized treatment approach, assessing the risks of developing metastatic disease balanced against the treatment toxicity and efficacy. Currently, there are several acceptable treatment options: (1) local salvage options, which provide last chance for possible cure (salvage radiation therapy for BCR after RP and salvage prostatectomy in selected patients after RT); (2) close surveillance; (3) intermittent or continuous ADT; and (4) clinical trials.

PATIENT SELECTION AND TIMING OF THERAPY

ADT is a standard systemic therapy for BCR patients who are not candidates for or who have failed or refused salvage treatment. Although ADT overall is manageable, it has a variety of side effects, mostly affecting quality of life as well as having an impact on other morbidities, such as sarcopenia, cardiovascular disease, osteoporosis, and diabetes.

The critical yet still somewhat ambiguous question for patients with BCR is whether earlier ADT treatment is beneficial for BCR patients. Retrospective studies demonstrated that early ADT has no significant effect on OS because it may decrease PCSM but increases non–PCSM.[10–12] Garcia-Albeniz and colleagues[13] presented a retrospective study of 2012 BCR patients from CaPSURE registry at the 2014 annual American Society of Clinical Oncology meeting. Patients who underwent immediate ADT (within 3 months of relapse) had no significant advantage in PCSM (hazard ratio [HR] 1.15) and all-cause mortality (HR 0.94). The immediate ADT arm had an estimated 5-year OS rate of 85.1% whereas the deferred ADT arm (>2 years after relapse) had 87.2%. The estimated 10-year OS was 71.6% in both arms, again demonstrating no significant advantage of early ADT treatment.[13] More

recently, an analysis of 2 phase 3 trials evaluating early ADT in BCR was presented together in a pre-planned analysis of 339 patients who were prospectively evaluated. Although an initial publication (including some metastatic patients who were castration sensitive) suggested a benefit of ADT, the studies demonstrated that early ADT did not improve survival in this BCR population.[14,15]

One of the key prognostic markers for potentially predicting outcomes in patients with BCR is PSA doubling time (PSADT), because several studies have reported the association between PSADT and risk of disease progression and development of metastatic disease, PCSM, and all-cause mortality.[3,16,17] Klayton and colleagues[18] analyzed 432 BCR patients treated with 3-dimensional conformal radiotherapy or intensity-modulated radiotherapy from 1989 to 2005 and demonstrated that PSADT is a significant predictor of prostate cancer–specific survival. Early initiation of ADT in patients with PSADT less than 6 months was significantly associated with improved prostate cancer–specific survival, although the survival benefit was less apparent in patients with longer PSADT.[18] Another retrospective study of 8669 patients with prostate cancer treated with RT (5918 patients) or RP (2751 patients) found that a PSADT less than 3 months also was significantly associated with PCSM.[16] Choueiri and colleagues[19] reported a retrospective study of 3071 prostate cancer patients at Duke University (between 1988 and 2008) who underwent RP. After a median follow-up of 7.4 years, BCR was diagnosed in 17.8% patients and 14.8% had died of all causes. The median follow-up after PSA failure was 11.2 years. In patients with BCR, a PSADT less than 6 months was associated with a significantly increased risk of overall death from any cause (HR 1.55).[19] D'Amico and colleagues[16] have reported that patients with PSADT greater than 15 months after RP are at minimal risk for prostate cancer metastasis or PCSM, whereas those with a PSADT of 3 months or less are at very high risk. In addition to these studies, a natural history study of 1997 patients who underwent RP and were followed for a mean of 5.3 years was reported by Pound and colleagues.[8] They found that 315 patients (15%) developed BCR, and 103 patients (34%) were not treated with immediate ADT developed metastatic disease. Those who developed metastatic disease more rapidly had PSADT less than 10 months, a Gleason score of greater than or equal to 8, and BCR onset within 2 years after RP.

For patients and providers who elect to treat BCR with ADT, questions remain about the type of ADT and treatment duration. Limited data exist on the utility of monotherapy with gonadotropin-releasing hormone agonist or antagonist, antiandrogens, or combined androgen blockade. Intermittent ADT (8 months of ADT followed by treatment break until PSA >10 ng/mL) is the preferred option for many clinicians and is based on results of a large randomized phase III, noninferiority study randomly assigning 1386 men with BCR after RT to intermittent or continuous ADT. Intermittent ADT was noninferior (HR 1.02; 95% CI, 0.86–1.21) and quality of life was significantly superior compared with the continuous ADT.[20]

THE ROLE OF IMMUNOTHERAPY IN PROSTATE CANCER

At this point, the role for immunotherapy in prostate cancer is somewhat limited compared with other genitourinary malignancies, such as urothelial cancer and renal cell cancer. Furthermore, most immunotherapy trials have been conducted in men with advanced prostate cancer who already have progressed on ADT, that is, metastatic castration–resistant prostate cancer (mCRPC). In a phase 3 study, sipuleucel-T showed a survival benefit in minimally symptomatic men with mCRPC.[21] Sipuleucel-T is activated cellular therapy (or vaccine) that is derived from a patient's own peripheral blood mononuclear cells (PBMCs). Once removed from a patient's circulation using apheresis, these PBMCs are exposed to the prostate cancer antigen prostatic acid phosphatase (PAP) as well as the cytokine granulocyte-macrophage colony-stimulating factor (GM-CSF) for approximately 48 hours ex vivo. The cells then are reinfused back into the patient every 2 weeks for total of 3 doses.

Despite these findings, the role of sipuleucel-T has been limited for several reasons. First and foremost, the clinical trial demonstrating an improvement in OS did not show a short-term improvement in progression-free survival (PFS). These findings predated the robust clinical development of checkpoint inhibitors; thus, practitioners were not accustomed to the potential delayed clinical impact seen with immune-based therapies. This led to some degree of discomfort using a therapy that showed an OS benefit without a benefit in PFS. This was complicated only further by the lack of substantial PSA declines, even though the Prostate Cancer Clinical Trials Working Group (PCWG) guidelines state that PSA responses should not be used to determine clinical benefit in mCRPC.[22] Thus, although sipuleucel-T remains available today, the treatment by providers is limited based at least partially on dogma

that has roots before the modern immune-oncology era as well as subsequent approvals of more conventional antiandrogens like enzalutamide and abiraterone.

Immune checkpoint inhibitors have a limited role in subpopulations of mCRPC patients. Patients with specific genetic mutations, such as microsatellite instability and CDK12 inactivation[23,24] (seen in approximately 5%–10% of prostate cancer patients), appear to respond to PD-1 and PD-L1 inhibition. Response rates to those forms of immunotherapies in mCRPC, however, are approximately 50% based on a small amount of data available thus far. In the largest experience reported to date of PD-1/PD-L1 inhibition, pembrolizumab was reported to have a minimal impact in an unselected population.[25]

Ipilimumab, an anti–CTLA-4 antibody, has been evaluated in 2 large phase 3 trials in mCRPC, both before and after chemotherapy. The first trial, done in the more advanced, postchemotherapy setting after 8-Gy radiotherapy to 1 site of metastatic disease, was nearly positive for its OS endpoint, 11.2 months versus 10.0 months with placebo (HR 0.85; $P = 0.053$).[26] These findings raised hopes for a concurrent trial being done in patients who were chemotherapy-naïve and thus potentially had more time to benefit from an immune-based therapy. This trial failed, however, to meet its primary endpoint of OS.[27] These findings, coupled with the toxicity of anti–CTLA-4 inhibition, reduce enthusiasm for testing ipilimumab in patients with BCR.

RATIONALE FOR IMMUNOTHERAPY IN BIOCHEMICALLY RECURRENT PROSTATE CANCER

There are several potentially important biologic characteristics that differentiate the BCR patients compared with patients with advanced mCRPC, where several studies, including those with immune checkpoint inhibitors, have been negative[25–27] (**Table 1**). Patients with BCR have microscopic metastatic disease, not seen on conventional imaging. Thus, compared with patients with macroscopic tumors in advanced disease, it is likely that tumor-related immune suppression (possibly related to increased immunosuppressive cytokines) would be decreased.[28] Furthermore, those micrometastatic foci in BCR appear to be more likely present in lymph nodes as opposed to the bone microenvironment, where 90% of men with mCRPC have substantial disease burden.[29] Biologically speaking, the lymph node may be more conducive to an immune response than the metastatic bone microenvironment.[30]

Table 1
Important biologic differences between patients with biochemically recurrent prostate cancer and metastatic castration–resistant prostate cancer

	Biochemically Recurrent Prostate Cancer	Metastatic Castration–Resistant Prostate Cancer
Testosterone levels	Normal physiologic levels	Castrate levels of testosterone
Predominant Sites of Disease	Lymph nodes (based on early PET imaging)	Bone
Tumor Burden	Minimal—not seen on conventional CT or Tc99 bone scan	Variable—but substantial enough to be seen on conventional imaging

Finally, the impact of long-term testosterone suppression and androgen receptor–targeted therapies on the immune microenvironment has been inadequately studied, although studies of immune checkpoint inhibitors in lung cancer have suggested that men may respond better than women.[31] Furthermore, castration may have an impact on the immune microenvironment by increasing suppressive factors, such as myeloid-derived suppressor cells.[32] Although it remains unclear if any of these factors truly potentiate immunotherapy in BCR over mCRPC, these could be reasons why clinical outcomes with immunotherapy may be different in BCR compared with advanced prostate cancer.

Another key aspect for any therapy in BCR is toxicity. ADT is already available and, although it has unclear benefits, the short-term impact on PSA usually is positive and often allays anxiety in this population of men with rising PSA values. For many BCR patients, the limiting aspect of ADT is toxicity. This highlights an important treatment consideration for men with BCR because these patients have no symptoms from their disease. As data from cancer prevention trials show, patients without symptoms often are reluctant to take therapies that have substantial toxicity.[33,34] Thus, relative to ADT or chemotherapy, immunotherapy (especially vaccine-based strategies) often carries minimal side effects and thus is more likely to be acceptable in the population.

Although ADT has not been shown to improve survival in this population, nonhormonal treatments that can alter PSADT may delay the morbidity associated with the development and treatment of metastatic disease, as reported by a retrospective study of BCR patients who were enrolled in trials at Johns Hopkins University.[35] For 146 patients treated in 4 clinical trials, there was a benefit when therapies were able to improve PSA kinetics 6 months after therapy. For patients who had prolongation of PSADT, the metastasis-free survival (MFS) was 63.5 months compared with 28.9 months in those whose PSADT was unchanged.

These findings could highlight the potential opportunity and benefits for immunotherapy in this population as means to delay metastatic progression and perhaps improve long-term outcomes. Data from previous studies, including sipuleucel-T, suggest that immunotherapy in prostate cancer may slow the growth rate of the disease. This could explain why sipuleucel-T demonstrated a survival advantage in a phase 3 study in mCRPC without showing a short-term benefit in PFS or PSA.[21,36] This benefit may be especially valuable in BCR patients who may live a decade or more whereas mCRPC patients may progress in months and die within years. The potential to allow time for an immune response to develop may be critical for strategies that have an impact on the immune microenvironment beyond simple immune checkpoint inhibition.

SELECTED STUDIES OF IMMUNOTHERAPY IN BIOCHEMICALLY RECURRENT PROSTATE CANCER

Several trials previously have explored the potential role of immunotherapy in BCR prostate cancer (**Table 2**). Therapeutic cancer vaccines generally have minimal toxicity and thus they are viable candidates for the asymptomatic men with BCR. Several studies have explored the potential role for therapeutic cancer vaccines of having an impact on prostate cancer in this disease state, often paired with ADT.

Sipuleucel-T was administered in patients with BCR in a randomized trial in patients who developed a rising PSA after RP within 2 years after surgery.[37] This multicenter trial randomized patients in a 2:1 fashion to either placebo or sipuleucel-T, administered at what has become the standard schedule of infusions, at weeks 0, 2, and 4. ADT was given prior to sipuleucel-T by 3 months to

Table 2
Selected trials of immunotherapy in biochemically recurrent prostate cancer

Treatment	Design and Key Results	Citation
Sipuleucel-T	• Patients: rising PSA within 2 y after surgery • ADT followed by sipuleucel-T • Sipuleucel-T was associated with improved PSADT after testosterone recovery	Beer et al,[37] 2011
Sipuleucel-T	• Patients: PSADT less than or equal to 12 mo • Evaluated sequence of ADT and sipuleucel-T • Better immune responses seen with sipuleucel-T followed by ADT but no difference in PSA recovery	Antonarakis et al,[38] 2017
PROSTVAC	• PROSTVAC followed by ADT • PROSTVAC alone improved PSADT from 5.3 mo to 7.7 mo • PROSTVAC + ADT resulted in complete responses in 20 of 27 patients (74%)	DiPaola et al,[40] 2015
PROSTVAC	• Prostvac in patients with PSADT 5–15 mo • Subset of patients had delayed but sustained PSA declines (range 10%–99%)	Madan et al,[43] 2018
TARP vaccine	• Patients with BCR and HLA-A*0201 • Patients treated with vaccine had slowing of slope log(PSA) in 72% of patients at 24 wk	Wood et al,[46] 2016
pTVG-HP	• Patients with BCR and a PSADT <12 mo • No difference in PSADT or MFS vs GM-CSF control • Improvements seen in 23% of vaccine patients on NaF PET imaging	McNeel et al,[49] 2019

Data from Refs.[37,38,40,43,46,49]

4 months. The primary endpoint of the trial was time to biochemical failure, but the study did not show a clear impact of sipuleucel-T (18 months) relative to the control group (15.4 months; HR 0.936; $P = .737$). Despite these findings, sipuleucel-T had an impact on increasing (ie, improving) PSADT in patients after testosterone recovery of 48%, or 155 days versus 105 days ($P = .038$).

A subsequent trial using sipuleucel-T sequenced with ADT evaluated sequences of ADT before and after sipuleucel-T in BCR patients. Although the study found no difference in mean time of PSA recurrence between the sequences, there were greater immune responses (antigen-specific T-cell proliferation and humoral responses) among patients who received vaccine followed by ADT. These data perhaps suggest an optimal sequence of immunotherapy when paired with ADT in BCR.[38]

PROSTVAC is a viral vector–based immunotherapy that is composed of 2 recombinant viral vectors, each encoding transgenes for PSA, and a triad of costimulatory molecules (B7.1, ICAM-1, and LFA-3). PROSTVAC initially was studied in a phase I trial, showing safety and feasibility in 15 patients who received recombinant fowlpox-PSA (triad of costimulatory molecules alone or recombinant vaccinia-PSA/triad of costimulatory molecules followed by recombinant fowlpox-PSA/triad of costimulatory molecules on a prime and boost schedule with or without recombinant GM-CSF protein or recombinant fowlpox- GM-CSF vector).[39] A further phase II trial in the form of E9802 was launched with an aim of determining safety and effectiveness of PROSTVAC-V (vaccinia)/TRICOM on cycle 1 followed by PROSTVAC-F (fowlpox)/triad of costimulatory moleculaes (TRICOM) for subsequent cycles in combination with GM-CSF as a first step followed by additional ADT in step 2 in patients with PSA progression without visible metastasis.[40] The primary endpoint for step 1 was to characterize the PSA velocity but also to determine PSA progression at 6 months, and the endpoint for step 2 was to determine PSA response in combination with ADT. The trial results were promising, with a majority of patients, at 63% (25 of 40 patients in step 1), achieving PFS at 6 months with potential slowing of logarithmic PSA velocity translating to a delay in PSADT from 5.3 months to 7.7 months. Furthermore, there were complete responses in 20 patients of 27 patients (74%; 90% CI, 57–87) who were eligible to be evaluated for step 2 (the additional ADT arm). The use of PROSTVAC was supported in other populations of prostate cancer, including that of mCRPC, where phase II data showed an 8.5-month improvement in OS and 44% reduction in the risk of death,[41] although a follow-up phase III trial of PROSTVAC in asymptomatic and minimally symptomatic mCRPC patients unfortunately showed no improvement in OS.[42]

Another study of PROSTVAC in BCR evaluated patients with a PSADT between 5 months and 15 months and treated them with 6 months of PROSTVAC and no ADT compared with surveillance. Preliminary data indicated that a subpopulation of patients (approximately 20%) had delayed PSA declines after an initial rise. The decline often occurred after completing vaccine and while on no ADT or additional therapy. Declines ranged from 10% to 99%, and many declines were sustained for many months. These data highlight the potential to for late effects in this population that otherwise would be surveilled.[43]

T-cell receptor alternate reading frame protein (TARP) is a novel immunogenic protein that is abundantly expressed by prostate cancer epithelial cells, initially described in 1999,[44] that is up-regulated by androgens and variably expressed in different states, including in the aggressive prostate cancers, metastatic prostate cancer,[45] and both hormone-sensitive and castration-resistant disease, making it an attractive antigenic target for prostate cancer vaccine therapy. A first-in-human pilot study involved 41 patients with hormone-sensitive BCR prostate cancer with HLA-A*0201 who were randomized in a 1:1 ratio to either cohort A, where patients received 1 mg of each peptide emulsified together with GM-CSF in Montanide ISA51VG and GM-CSF given subcutaneously, or cohort B patients, who were given autologous dendritic cells pulsed with each peptide plus keyhole limpet hemocyanin intradermally.[46] The study aimed at determining safety of the vaccine approach and measuring the immunogenicity of the TARP peptide vaccination because it has an impact on the PSA velocity (as expressed as slope log[PSA]) or the PSADT and tumor growths. Given a schedule of every 3 weeks for a total of 5 vaccinations with an optional sixth dose of vaccine at 36 weeks, the study showed a majority of patients had a statistically significant slowing in the postvaccination slope log(PSA) (equivalent to an increase/lengthening in PSADT), with declines seen in 72% of patients reaching 24 weeks and 74% reaching 48 weeks ($P = .0012$ and $P = .0004$, respectively, for comparison of overall changes in slope log [PSA]). Although TARP vaccination also showed a 50% decrease in median tumor growth rate, only 15% of patients exhibited decrease in serum PSA levels.

PAP has been shown to be an effective target for sipuleucel-T and there are additional strategies to target PAP. Alternatives, such as using a DNA vaccine encoding PAP that can elicit antigen-specific $CD8^+$ T cells, were studied in early phase I/II trials utilizing DNA vaccine (pTVG-HP [MVI-816]) that encodes PAP in men with non-mCRPC (nmCRPC); 22 patients were enrolled in this study and 3 (14%) developed PAP-specific interferon gamma–secreting $CD8^+$ T cells.[47] Another trial in nmCRPC patients established safety and showed early potential of a plasmid DNA vaccine. Vaccines are given as 6 injections at 2-week intervals and then either quarterly (arm 1) or as determined by multiparameter immune monitoring (arm 2). At 2 years, 6 of 16 patients (38%) remained metastasis-free.[48] A phase II trial, that utilized the same DNA vaccine, enrolled 99 patients with hormone-sensitive prostate cancer and PSADT of less than 12 months, with treatment either with pTVG-HP coadministered intradermally, with 200-mg GM-CSF, or 200-mg GM-CSF alone 6 times biweekly and then quarterly for 2 years.[49] The primary endpoint was 2-year MFS, which showed no difference between the study arms (41.8% vaccine vs 42.3%, respectively; $P = .97$). Changes in PSADT and median MFS were not different between study arms (18.9 months vs 18.3 months, respectively; HR 1.6; $P = .13$). Decreases in standardized uptake value were seen on sodium fluoride (NaF) PET/CT scan in 23% of vaccine patients versus increases in 50% of controls ($P = .07$).

Selected Current Trials of Immunotherapy in Biochemically Recurrent Prostate Cancer

Although prostate cancer is generally thought to be non-responsive to immune checkpoint inhibitors because of low tumor mutational burden (TMB) and limited T cell immune infiltration, several ongoing studies are evaluating immune checkpoint inhibitors based on immune potential synergies or patient selection.[50] Several studies, however, have reported notable expression of PD-L1, which is up-regulated by interferon-gamma signaling,[51,52] in primary prostate cancer specimens (up to approximately 60%) and CRPC tissue (up to approximately 20%), implying active inflammatory signaling. Inflamed tumors are associated with particularly high risk of recurrence.[52] In a study of RP specimens, PD-L1 expression in greater than or equal to 1% of tumor cells ranged from 13.8% in tumors of any grade to 26.5% of Gleason score 8 to 10 tumors.[53] Moreover, PD-L1 expression was associated with CD8$^+$ T-cell infiltration. This is remarkably similar to the 17% of primary prostate cancers in a separate study that were found to have a DNA damage repair and inflammation gene expression signature predictive of Stimulator of interferon genes (STING) activation as well as increased risk of BCR.[54]

Thus, 1 hypothesis is that patients with BCR could be particularly enriched for having immunogenic tumors and that checkpoint inhibition could be more effective in the micrometastatic and precastration settings. This is being tested in a phase 2 study of nivolumab monotherapy for patients with high-risk BCR prostate cancer based on a PSADT of less than 10 months (NCT03637543). Diagnostic core biopsies (for patients who received primary radiation) or prostatectomy specimens are assessed for tumor PD-L1 expression greater than or equal to 5% by the E1L3N clone, and patients then are assigned to a PD-L1–positive or PD-L1–negative cohort. Once enrolled, if patients experience PSA stabilization or responses, then they can continue to receive nivolumab for up to 2 years in the absence of progression to metastatic disease or unacceptable toxicity. Patients who have isolated PSA progression at 12 weeks can be continued on treatment at investigator's discretion if they are believed to be clinically benefitting (for example, if they experience decreased PSADT time) and have not demonstrated symptomatic or radiographic evidence of metastatic disease.

The primary endpoint is disease control, defined as PSA after 12 weeks of nivolumab that is less than 10% above baseline, or below baseline, and with no symptomatic/radiographic progression. This is more stringent than the PCWG3 definition, which considers PSA progression to be a rise of at least 25% of baseline, because if patients enter the study with a 10-month PSADT, then they would be expected to have a 23% increase in PSA without any intervention.

A variety of planned correlative studies will allow assessment of tumor-based and blood-based biomarkers, including genomics, gene expression, immune tumor microenvironment, T-cell clonality, and soluble biomarkers. These also will help advance understanding of additional mechanisms of resistance to checkpoint inhibition to form the basis for future trials in this space.

Given the promising results of this trial in advanced disease, the combination of pTVG-HP with PD-1 blockade pembrolizumab in patients with castration-sensitive, PSA-recurrent prostate cancer currently is under way (NCT02499835). The combination offers a better concurrent and synergistic approach, rather than a sequential approach, as seen in a combination trial.[55] This therapeutic strategy serves to capitalize on improving antineoplastic activity of the DNA vaccine theoretically by increasing up-regulation and T-cell activation at the time of PD-1 blockade[56] and that PD-1–regulated T-cell activation also was seen in patients treated with a DNA vaccine encoding PAP.[57]

A similar combination strategy is being evaluated at the National Cancer Institute, building on the late PSA declines seen with PROSTVAC alone in BCR patients.[43] In this follow-up study, patients will be surveilled for 4 months before starting multiple vaccines (PROSTVAC and the CV-301 targeting CEA/MUC1). Then, after 4 months of both vaccines, patients will be treated with bintrafusp alfa, a bifunctional fusion protein targeting transforming growth factor β and PD-L1. Immune correlates will evaluate the impact of multiple vaccines in this population compared with one in the previous study and evaluate changes after bintrafusp alfa is added (NCT03315871).

The Future Perspective of Biochemically Recurrent Prostate Cancer in the Age of Modern Imaging

CT scans are considered standard for staging of many solid tumors, including prostate cancer. Although they are not perfect and can miss nodal metastases if size is less than 1.5 cm, they are effective for evaluation of visceral and bone metastases. The gold standard for detection of bone metastases remains Tc99 bone scan; however, its utility is limited in BCR patients with lower PSA values. Both CT and Tc99 bone scans have been utilized for decades in BCR patients; however, the question is whether earlier identification of metastatic disease can influence treatment decisions.

Many efforts have been made to develop novel imaging modalities. One of the most commonly used novel imaging tools is fludeoxyglucose F 18–PET scan; however, this scan has limited sensitivity for detection of lymph node metastases.[58] The most promising novel imaging modalities for the BCR include choline C 11–PET (choline metabolism is impaired in prostate cancer), ^{68}Ga/^{18}F–prostate-specific membrane antigen (transmembrane protein highly expressed in prostate cancer), and anti–fluorocyclobutane F 18–1-carboxylic acid (Axumin) a synthetic L-leucine analog that demonstrates uptake in prostate cancer. Those new modalities have entered into clinical practice, with higher detection of metastatic disease at low PSA levels; however, more prospective studies are needed to define utility of novel scans in making treatment decisions.[58]

Although one point of view may suggest that modern imaging studies will make the disease state of BCR obsolete, that probably is a limited perspective. Some proponents of modern imaging in BCR may suggest that once metastatic sites are identified, the patients have de facto metastatic castration–sensitive disease and thus lifelong ADT is indicated along with docetaxel or antiandrogen therapy. But none of the trials in metastatic castration–sensitive prostate cancer allowed molecular or PET imaging to be the sole mechanism to detect metastatic disease.[59–61] In addition, these studies predominantly evaluated newly diagnosed patients and less frequently in patients with disease recurrence. Furthermore, the natural history of BCR is so variable that over-treatment of patients with BCR would be inevitable. It is unclear if patients would live longer starting ADT for PET-positive metastatic disease compared with waiting until conventional imaging detects their cancer. The toxicity would be magnified if chemotherapy or antiandrogens are added, not to mention the financial ramifications of such choices for the more than 25,000 men a year with BCR.

The alternative strategy would be to treat oligometastatic PET-positive sites in patients with BCR (based on conventional imaging). Although is increasingly is being done in the community, often with the goal of cure, emerging data suggest that it is most effective in patients with limited sites of disease.[62] Furthermore, when different modern (ie, PET) strategies are compared, the metastatic sites do not always overlap.[63] Thus, even with modern imaging, technology still may limit the oligometastatic sites that could be seen and then targeted.

The evolution of modern imaging actually may open up a new therapeutic front in prostate cancer in the BCR space or facilitate patient selection for treatment escalation/de-escalation. The terms may be different (eg, PET-positive disease or PET metastatic, castration sensitive) but once imaging can detect the disease, one of the greatest constraints on large-scale therapeutic development in BCR will have been removed—a lack of an intermediate endpoint that can demonstrate efficacy. All trials in BCR, whether or not they include immunotherapy, now should require molecular imaging to define their clinical impact beyond just PSA values or PSA kinetics. If immunotherapy strategies can demonstrate delayed progression on modern imaging or even improvements on scans, then that could certainly open the door to clinical development, applying the same logic that has been utilized in developing the ICECaP approach for MFS as an endpoint.[64] In this way, modern imaging is not the end of BCR; it actually opens a new frontier in prostate cancer research, much like CHAARTED and STAMPEDE did with metastatic, castration-sensitive disease. In some ways, this disease state will be more complicated because treatments will be required to balance long-ranging, life-altering impact with short-term effects on quality of life. If immunotherapy strategies can have an impact on the disease in this space (perhaps because of smaller tumor burden, anatomic location, or less castration-related immune suppression) and demonstrate that impact on modern imaging, they may have advantages in this asymptomatic population compared with ADT-centric regimens with immediate and long-term side effects. This is a unique time in prostate cancer, where imaging and immunotherapy may evolve symbiotically in the BCR population to better define how both can be used in the future.

REFERENCES

1. Siegel RL, Miller KD, Jemal A. Cancer statistics, 2020. CA Cancer J Clin 2020;70(1):7–30.
2. Roehl KA, Han M, Ramos CG, et al. Cancer progression and survival rates following anatomical radical retropubic prostatectomy in 3,478 consecutive patients: long-term results. J Urol 2004;172(3):910–4.
3. Freedland SJ, Humphreys EB, Mangold LA, et al. Risk of prostate cancer-specific mortality following biochemical recurrence after radical prostatectomy. JAMA 2005;294(4):433–9.
4. Freedland SJ, Humphreys EB, Mangold LA, et al. Death in patients with recurrent prostate cancer after radical prostatectomy: prostate-specific antigen doubling time subgroups and their associated contributions to all-cause mortality. J Clin Oncol 2007; 25(13):1765–71.
5. Cookson MS, Aus G, Burnett AL, et al. Variation in the definition of biochemical recurrence in patients treated for localized prostate cancer: the American Urological Association Prostate Guidelines for Localized Prostate Cancer Update Panel report and recommendations for a standard in the reporting of surgical outcomes. J Urol 2007;177(2):540–5.
6. Abramowitz MC, Li T, Buyyounouski MK, et al. The Phoenix definition of biochemical failure predicts for overall survival in patients with prostate cancer. Cancer 2008;112(1):55–60.
7. Horwitz EM, Thames HD, Kuban DA, et al. Definitions of biochemical failure that best predict clinical failure in patients with prostate cancer treated with external beam radiation alone: a multi-institutional pooled analysis. J Urol 2005;173(3):797–802.
8. Pound CR, Partin AW, Eisenberger MA, et al. Natural history of progression after PSA elevation following radical prostatectomy. JAMA 1999;281(17):1591–7.
9. Jhaveri FM, Zippe CD, Klein EA, et al. Biochemical failure does not predict overall survival after radical prostatectomy for localized prostate cancer: 10-year results. Urology 1999;54(5):884–90.
10. Loblaw DA, Virgo KS, Nam R, et al. Initial hormonal management of androgen-sensitive metastatic, recurrent, or progressive prostate cancer: 2007 update of an American Society of Clinical Oncology Practice guideline. J Clin Oncol 2007;25(12):1596–605.
11. Immediate versus deferred treatment for advanced prostatic cancer: initial results of the Medical Research Council Trial. The Medical Research Council Prostate Cancer Working Party Investigators Group. Br J Urol 1997;79(2):235–46.
12. Kirk D. Timing and choice of androgen ablation. Prostate Cancer Prostatic Dis 2004;7(3):217–22.
13. X Garcia-Albeniz JMC, Alan TP, Logan RW, et al. Immediate versus deferred initiation of androgen deprivation therapy in prostate cancer patients with PSA-only relapse. ASCO Annual Meeting. Chicago. J Clin Oncol 2014;32:5s (suppl; abstr 5003). Available at: https://meetinglibrary.asco.org/record/92302/abstract.
14. Duchesne GM, Woo HH, Bassett JK, et al. Timing of androgen-deprivation therapy in patients with prostate cancer with a rising PSA (TROG 03.06 and VCOG PR 01-03 [TOAD]): a randomised, multicentre, non-blinded, phase 3 trial. Lancet Oncol 2016;17(6):727–37.
15. Loblaw A, Bassett J, D'Este C, et al. Timing of androgen deprivation therapy for prostate cancer patients after radiation: Planned combined analysis of two randomized phase 3 trials. J Clin Oncol 2018;36(15_suppl):5018.
16. D'Amico AV, Moul JW, Carroll PR, et al. Surrogate end point for prostate cancer-specific mortality after radical prostatectomy or radiation therapy. J Natl Cancer Inst 2003;95(18):1376–83.
17. Smith MR, Kabbinavar F, Saad F, et al. Natural history of rising serum prostate-specific antigen in men with castrate nonmetastatic prostate cancer. J Clin Oncol 2005;23(13):2918–25.
18. Klayton TL, Ruth K, Buyyounouski MK, et al. Prostate-specific antigen doubling time predicts the development of distant metastases for patients who fail 3-dimensional conformal radiotherapy or intensity modulated radiation therapy using the Phoenix definition. Pract Radiat Oncol 2011;1(4):235–42.
19. Choueiri TK, Chen MH, D'Amico AV, et al. Impact of postoperative prostate-specific antigen disease recurrence and the use of salvage therapy on the risk of death. Cancer 2010;116(8):1887–92.
20. Crook JM, O'Callaghan CJ, Duncan G, et al. Intermittent androgen suppression for rising PSA level after radiotherapy. N Engl J Med 2012;367(10):895–903.
21. Kantoff PW, Higano CS, Shore ND, et al. Sipuleucel-T immunotherapy for castration-resistant prostate cancer. N Engl J Med 2010;363(5):411–22.
22. Scher HI, Halabi S, Tannock I, et al. Design and end points of clinical trials for patients with progressive prostate cancer and castrate levels of testosterone: recommendations of the Prostate Cancer Clinical Trials Working Group. J Clin Oncol 2008;26(7):1148–59.
23. Graham LS, Montgomery B, Cheng HH, et al. Mismatch repair deficiency in metastatic prostate cancer: Response to PD-1 blockade and standard therapies. PLoS One 2020;15(5):e0233260.
24. Reimers MA, Yip SM, Zhang L, et al. Clinical outcomes in cyclin-dependent kinase 12 mutant advanced prostate cancer. Eur Urol 2020;77(3):333–41.
25. Antonarakis ES, Piulats JM, Gross-Goupil M, et al. Pembrolizumab for treatment-refractory metastatic castration-resistant prostate cancer: multicohort,

open-label phase II KEYNOTE-199 study. J Clin Oncol 2020;38(5):395–405.

26. Kwon ED, Drake CG, Scher HI, et al. Ipilimumab versus placebo after radiotherapy in patients with metastatic castration-resistant prostate cancer that had progressed after docetaxel chemotherapy (CA184-043): a multicentre, randomised, double-blind, phase 3 trial. Lancet Oncol 2014;15(7):700–12.

27. Beer TM, Kwon ED, Drake CG, et al. Randomized, double-blind, phase III trial of ipilimumab versus placebo in asymptomatic or minimally symptomatic patients with metastatic chemotherapy-naive castration-resistant prostate cancer. J Clin Oncol 2017;35(1):40–7.

28. Silvestri I, Cattarino S, Agliano AM, et al. Beyond the immune suppression: the immunotherapy in prostate cancer. Biomed Res Int 2015;2015:794968.

29. Roach PJ, Francis R, Emmett L, et al. The Impact of (68)Ga-PSMA PET/CT on management intent in prostate cancer: results of an australian prospective multicenter study. J Nucl Med 2018;59(1):82–8.

30. Jiao S, Subudhi SK, Aparicio A, et al. Differences in tumor microenvironment dictate t helper lineage polarization and response to immune checkpoint therapy. Cell 2019;179(5):1177–1190 e13.

31. Wang C, Qiao W, Jiang Y, et al. Effect of sex on the efficacy of patients receiving immune checkpoint inhibitors in advanced non-small cell lung cancer. Cancer Med 2019;8(8):4023–31.

32. Calcinotto A, Spataro C, Zagato E, et al. IL-23 secreted by myeloid cells drives castration-resistant prostate cancer. Nature 2018;559(7714):363.

33. Ropka ME, Keim J, Philbrick JT. Patient decisions about breast cancer chemoprevention: a systematic review and meta-analysis. J Clin Oncol 2010;28(18):3090–5.

34. Dunn BK, Kramer BS. Cancer prevention: lessons learned and future directions. Trends Cancer 2016;2(12):713–22.

35. Antonarakis ES, Zahurak ML, Lin J, et al. Changes in PSA kinetics predict metastasis- free survival in men with PSA-recurrent prostate cancer treated with nonhormonal agents: combined analysis of 4 phase II trials. Cancer 2012;118(6):1533–42.

36. Madan RA, Gulley JL, Fojo T, et al. Therapeutic cancer vaccines in prostate cancer: the paradox of improved survival without changes in time to progression. Oncologist 2010;15(9):969–75.

37. Beer TM, Bernstein GT, Corman JM, et al. Randomized trial of autologous cellular immunotherapy with sipuleucel-T in androgen-dependent prostate cancer. Clin Cancer Res 2011;17(13):4558–67.

38. Antonarakis ES, Kibel AS, Yu EY, et al. Sequencing of sipuleucel-t and androgen deprivation therapy in men with hormone-sensitive biochemically recurrent prostate cancer: a phase II randomized trial. Clin Cancer Res 2017;23(10):2451–9.

39. Arlen PM, Skarupa L, Pazdur M, et al. Clinical safety of a viral vector based prostate cancer vaccine strategy. J Urol 2007;178(4 Pt 1):1515–20.

40. DiPaola RS, Chen YH, Bubley GJ, et al. A national multicenter phase 2 study of prostate-specific antigen (PSA) pox virus vaccine with sequential androgen ablation therapy in patients with PSA progression: ECOG 9802. Eur Urol 2015;68(3):365–71.

41. Kantoff PW, Schuetz TJ, Blumenstein BA, et al. Overall survival analysis of a phase II randomized controlled trial of a Poxviral-based PSA-targeted immunotherapy in metastatic castration-resistant prostate cancer. J Clin Oncol 2010;28(7):1099–105.

42. Gulley JL, Borre M, Vogelzang NJ, et al. Phase III Trial of PROSTVAC in asymptomatic or minimally symptomatic metastatic castration-resistant prostate cancer. J Clin Oncol 2019;37(13):1051–61.

43. Madan RA, Karzai F, Bilusic M, et al. Immunotherapy for biochemically recurrent prostate cancer. J Clin Oncol 2018;36(6_suppl):215.

44. Essand M, Vasmatzis G, Brinkmann U, et al. High expression of a specific T-cell receptor gamma transcript in epithelial cells of the prostate. Proc Natl Acad Sci U S A 1999;96(16):9287–92.

45. Varambally S, Yu J, Laxman B, et al. Integrative genomic and proteomic analysis of prostate cancer reveals signatures of metastatic progression. Cancer Cell 2005;8(5):393–406.

46. Wood LV, Fojo A, Roberson BD, et al. TARP vaccination is associated with slowing in PSA velocity and decreasing tumor growth rates in patients with Stage D0 prostate cancer. Oncoimmunology 2016;5(8):e1197459.

47. McNeel DG, Dunphy EJ, Davies JG, et al. Safety and immunological efficacy of a DNA vaccine encoding prostatic acid phosphatase in patients with stage D0 prostate cancer. J Clin Oncol 2009;27(25):4047–54.

48. McNeel DG, Becker JT, Eickhoff JC, et al. Real-time immune monitoring to guide plasmid DNA vaccination schedule targeting prostatic acid phosphatase in patients with castration-resistant prostate cancer. Clin Cancer Res 2014;20(14):3692–704.

49. McNeel DG, Eickhoff JC, Johnson LE, et al. Phase II trial of a DNA vaccine encoding prostatic acid phosphatase (pTVG-HP [MVI-816]) in patients with progressive, nonmetastatic, castration-sensitive prostate cancer. J Clin Oncol 2019;37(36):3507–17.

50. Cristescu R, Mogg R, Ayers M, et al. Pan-tumor genomic biomarkers for PD-1 checkpoint blockade–based immunotherapy. Science 2018;362(6411):eaar3593.

51. Massari F, Ciccarese C, Calio A, et al. Magnitude of PD-1, PD-L1 and T lymphocyte expression on tissue from castration-resistant prostate adenocarcinoma:

an exploratory analysis. Target Oncol 2016;11(3):345–51.

52. Gevensleben H, Dietrich D, Golletz C, et al. The immune checkpoint regulator PD-L1 is highly expressed in aggressive primary prostate cancer. Clin Cancer Res 2016;22(8):1969–77.

53. Calagua C, Russo J, Sun Y, et al. Expression of PD-L1 in hormone-naive and treated prostate cancer patients receiving neoadjuvant abiraterone acetate plus prednisone and leuprolide. Clin Cancer Res 2017;23(22):6812–22.

54. Reilly E, McCavigan A, Walker SM, et al. Identification of a high-risk subgroup in primary prostate cancers presenting with targetable immune biology. Cancer Res 2018;78(13). Available at: https://cancerres.aacrjournals.org/content/78/13_Supplement/283.

55. McNeel DG, Eickhoff JC, Wargowski E, et al. Concurrent, but not sequential, PD-1 blockade with a DNA vaccine elicits anti-tumor responses in patients with metastatic, castration-resistant prostate cancer. Oncotarget 2018;9(39):25586–96.

56. Rekoske BT, Smith HA, Olson BM, et al. PD-1 or PD-L1 Blockade Restores Antitumor Efficacy Following SSX2 Epitope-Modified DNA Vaccine Immunization. Cancer Immunol Res 2015;3(8):946–55.

57. Rekoske BT, Olson BM, McNeel DG. Antitumor vaccination of prostate cancer patients elicits PD-1/PD-L1 regulated antigen-specific immune responses. Oncoimmunology 2016;5(6):e1165377.

58. Thoeny HC, Barbieri S, Froehlich JM, et al. Functional and targeted lymph node imaging in prostate cancer: current status and future challenges. Radiology 2017;285(3):728–43.

59. James ND, de Bono JS, Spears MR, et al. Abiraterone for prostate cancer not previously treated with hormone therapy. N Engl J Med 2017;377(4):338–51.

60. James ND, Sydes MR, Clarke NW, et al. Addition of docetaxel, zoledronic acid, or both to first-line long-term hormone therapy in prostate cancer (STAMPEDE): survival results from an adaptive, multiarm, multistage, platform randomised controlled trial. Lancet 2016;387(10024):1163–77.

61. Sweeney CJ, Chen YH, Carducci M, et al. Chemohormonal therapy in metastatic hormone-sensitive prostate cancer. N Engl J Med 2015;373(8):737–46.

62. Horn T, Kronke M, Rauscher I, et al. Single lesion on prostate-specific membrane antigen-ligand positron emission tomography and low prostate-specific antigen are prognostic factors for a favorable biochemical response to prostate-specific membrane antigen-targeted radioguided surgery in recurrent prostate cancer. Eur Urol 2019;76(4):517–23.

63. Harmon SA, Bergvall E, Mena E, et al. A prospective comparison of (18)F-Sodium Fluoride PET/CT and PSMA-Targeted (18)F-DCFBC PET/CT in metastatic prostate cancer. J Nucl Med 2018;59(11):1665–71.

64. Xie W, Regan MM, Buyse M, et al. Metastasis-free survival is a strong surrogate of overall survival in localized prostate cancer. J Clin Oncol 2017;35(27):3097–104.

Immunotherapy for Prostate Cancer: Treatments for the "Lethal" Phenotype

Susan F. Slovin, MD, PhD

KEYWORDS

- Immunotherapy • Prostate cancer • CDK12 • Sipuleucel T • Vaccines • Tumor microenvironment
- Checkpoint inhibitors

KEY POINTS

- Immunotherapy for prostate cancer has been limited by a "bland" or "cold" tumor microenvironment.
- Multiple mechanisms exist within the tumor microenvironment that inhibit infiltration of immune cells.
- Small cell/neuroendocrine prostate cancer represents a unique histologic phenotype that may occur de novo or may emerge following failure of androgen receptor signaling inhibitors.
- CDK12 mutated prostate cancer represents a unique group of tumors with limited sensitivity to checkpoint inhibitors.

INTRODUCTION

Prostate cancer remains the first solid tumor to demonstrate the overall survival (OS) of an autologous cellular therapy, Sipuleucel-T,[1] but despite its success, understanding why prostate cancer has been refractory to a wide range of subsequent immune platforms remains unclear. Modulations in prostate-specific antigen (PSA) have been demonstrated in several approaches,[2] but despite the success demonstrating survival benefit in a phase II trial of PROSTVAC (rilimogene galvacirepvec/rilimogene glafolivec) or F-PSA-TRICOM; PROSTVAC-V,[3] a viral-based immunotherapy consisting of a vaccinia virus and recombinant fowlpox virus given as a prime boost, no change in the biologic behavior of the cancer was seen. Both viruses encode modified forms of PSA, along with 3 costimulatory molecules, B7.1 (CD80), with intercellular adhesion molecule-1 (ICAM-1) and lymphocyte function-associated antigen-3 (LFA-3). The phase II study cited a prolonged median OS of 8.5 months versus placebo in men with castration-resistant prostate cancer (CRPC)[3]; the randomized phase III[4] trial did need not meet its primary endpoint of OS in men with castrated metastatic prostate cancer. In fact, at the third interim analysis, criteria for futility were made and the trial was stopped early. The study was designed to compare the superiority of PROSTVAC or PROSTVAC plus granulocyte/macrophage stimulating factor (GM-CSF), versus placebo. Although PROSTVAC induced T-cell–specific responses against PSA, as well as "cascade" antigens,[4,5] the immune response did not translate into clinical benefit.

TARGETING THE TUMOR MICROENVIRONMENT: A CHALLENGE?

It remains unclear whether the lack of response to multiple immunologic approaches is due to one cellular population or a combination of cytokines, cells, and inhibitory factors within this setting. Failures of immune-based therapies have been

Genitourinary Oncology Service, Department of Medicine, Sidney Kimmel Center for Prostate and Urologic Cancers, Memorial Sloan Kettering Cancer Center, 1275 York Avenue, New York, NY 10065, USA
E-mail address: slovins@mskcc.org

Urol Clin N Am 47 (2020) 469–474
https://doi.org/10.1016/j.ucl.2020.07.007
0094-0143/20/© 2020 Elsevier Inc. All rights reserved.

attributed to the "bland" or "cold" tumor microenvironment of prostate cancer due to lack of CD8 infiltration; inhibitory pathways such as adenosine,[6,7] or cellular populations such as myeloid-derived suppressor cells (MDSCs), colony stromal factor-1, or inhibitory macrophages have been closely studied. Multiple agents are currently in clinical trials targeting each of these pathways and cellular populations, but to date, no agent alone has met with success. More recently,[8] the inhibition of BRD4, member of the Bromodomain and ExtraTerminal (BET) family of bromodomain-containing proteins, has been shown to reduce levels of several target genes under androgen receptor (AR) control and can reduce tumor size in preclinical models. It has been postulated that in its role as a transcriptional regulator, BRD4 recruitment may participate in mediating AR and other oncogenic drivers such as MYC, but may have a potential role in immune regulations. As such, targeting BET bromodomains using a small molecule inhibitor has been shown to decrease PD-L1 expression and reduce tumor progression in prostate cancer models. It is likely that BET bromodomain inhibition works via increasing major histocompatibility complex class I expression, thereby increasing the immunogenicity of tumor cells. Furthermore, transcriptional profiling showed that BET bromodomain inhibition can modulate several networks that are involved in antigen processing and immune checkpoint molecules. Murine models treated with an inhibitor have demonstrated increased CD8/Treg populations, suggesting that there may be a role for using a bromodomain inhibitor along with a checkpoint inhibitor[8] in patients.

The greatest conundrum is why prostate cancers have been relatively resistant to checkpoint inhibitors. Although a phase I/II trial[9] using different doses of ipilimumab given alone or after radiation showed long-term benefit and even remission in a minority of patients, nevertheless 2 phase III trials,[10,11] both in early and late disease, respectively, did not meet their endpoints of survival, albeit, the "tail end" of the survival curve had patients with durable responses. Efforts to explain the lack of responsiveness of prostate cancer to this family of immune therapies remains an active area of study. Anecdotal case reports have suggested that some form of "immune modulation" can be seen if patients received enzalutamide first before receiving Sipuleucel-T, leading to a dramatic decline in PSA. In one case report,[12] a patient who had been in a clinical atrial and had received GM-CSF therapy resulting in "a saw-tooth like pattern of PSA declines during treatment,"

developed continued rises in PSA with development of castration-resistant disease to bone. He went on to treatment with enzalutamide with improvement in disease with declines in PSA but then developed rising PSAs. He then received Sipuleucel-T while continuing the enzalutamide and androgen-deprivation therapy, and after 6 months developed a marked decline in PSA to less than 0.05 that lasted for more than 1 year with regression of metastatic disease. This is clearly an unusual scenario, but raises the question of whether or not enzalutamide can enhance the effects not only of Sipuleucel-T but other immune-based therapies as well. That there was a delay in response may be attributed to an "immune-based mechanism" given prior results from Sipuleucel-T trials that suggested a robust increase in antigen-presenting cell (APC) upregulation. This patient had similar findings. Others[13,14] have demonstrated in small studies that patients with visceral metastases in the presence of genomic alterations such as BRCA 1,2 or MSI[hi] can respond robustly to pembrolizumab with long-term responses. This has led to a further inquiry as to how these agents may be used in patients with these genomic alterations and whether or not combinations with these agents may provide significant long-term benefits to patients who are otherwise refractory to standard androgen signaling inhibitors or chemotherapies. Antonarakis and colleagues,[15] in a multicohort Keynote 199 study, demonstrated that there may be benefit in a small but unique cohort of patients who received single-agent pembrolizumab, reinforcing our continued efforts to further define patients who may derive benefits from this therapeutic class of drugs.[16]

LETHAL PROSTATE CANCER: DOES IT EXIST AND CAN WE TREAT IT?

The term "lethal" has taken on many connotations, but in particular if usually viewed as a type of tumor that is aggressive at diagnosis or becomes aggressive following therapies, both with rapid progression to end-stage disease. More recently, it has come to be understood as a unique phenotype that has evolved following treatment with AR signaling inhibitors, such as enzalutamide and abiraterone, to unusual histologic subtypes as neuroendocrine prostate cancer.[17] Although adenocarcinoma remains the predominant histologic phenotype of prostate cancer and displays features suggestive of luminal prostate cells that are under androgen regulation, de novo small cell carcinoma of the prostate can appear that often bears similar histology to small cell carcinoma of the lung. This prostate variant can also appear later in the disease in the more treatment-refractory setting, often posing a challenge for the treating physician, as standard small cell chemotherapies do not provide durable responses. There has been a clinical lack of clarity with response to terminology, as small cell does not always mean neuroendocrine cancer, given that there are features that are either mixed to suggest that small cell and neuroendocrine or poorly differentiated prostate cancer can all align together. As such, the mixed histologic features within a continuum of histologic and behavioral evolution are encompassed under the umbrella of "neuroendocrine prostate cancer" with clear delineations regarding survival[17] (**Fig. 1**).

TREATING THE "LETHAL" PHENOTYPE BASED ON GENOMICS

Carreira and colleagues[18] suggest that there are unique tumor adaptations that may underlie resistance to repeated AR targeting in CRPC. As such, using targeted sequencing and computational approaches, they have systematically profiled genomic changes in a patient's tumor to demonstrate unique mutations in sites of metastatic disease that correspond to behavioral changes within the tumor and demonstrate clonal architectural heterogeneity at different stages of disease progression. This management paradigm may offer a means by which "lethality" can be identified early and treatments can be redirected to the more aggressive clones. Aggarwal and colleagues[19] systematically analyzed 202 patients of whom 148 had prior disease progression on abiraterone and/or enzalutamide and who underwent routine biopsies. The overall incidence of small cell neuroendocrine prostate cancer was 17% with AR amplification and protein expression noted in 67% and 75%, respectively. Detection of neuroendocrine cancer was associated with shortened OS among patients with prior AR-targeting therapy (hazard ratio 2.02; 95% confidence interval 1.07–3.82). A "transcriptional signature" was also developed and validated with greater than 90% accuracy and seems to indicate that this phenotype arises in the context of TP53 and RB1 aberration from adenocarcinoma under a selective process if not pressure of inhibition of the AR pathway.[20] They reported frequent loss of TP53 and/or RB1 at the genome level along with upregulation of E2F. Interestingly, DEK[21] was the highest overexpressed E2F1 target gene in the small cell/neuroendocrine cluster with prior implication into the progression to

this phenotype. Other transcriptional factors that have been documented into the progression into small cell/neuroendocrine prostate cancer include POU class 3 homeobox, FOX A2, ASCL1, and BRN2.

It is clear that from a behavioral and histologic standpoint, these "lethal" cancers may also have a unique response to immune agents. Wu and colleagues[22,23] have subsequently identified a unique subtype of prostate cancer that is associated with bi-allelic loss of CDK12 and is mutually exclusive with tumors driven by DNA repair deficiency in addition to ETS fusions and a variety of mutations in SPOP.[23] CDK12 is a cyclin-dependent kinase that forms a heterodimeric complex with cyclin K, its activating partner. Together, they regulate a variety of processes that regulate gene expression.[20] Using an integrative genomic analysis of 360 samples from patients with metastatic CRPC (mCRPC), samples that had CDK12 mutants were associated with increasing burden of neoantigens and increased infiltration and/or clonal expansion of tumor T cells. Interestingly, although most CDK12 mutants retained active AR, suggesting sensitivity to AR blocking or signaling inhibitors, they had a distinct expression signature that was characterized by increased gene fusions as well as increased gene fusion–induced neoantigen open reading frames. The latter served as rationale for exploring the susceptibility of those tumors with higher neoantigen burden could respond to alternative lines of therapy. Also in keeping with known susceptibility to checkpoint inhibitors, is an inflammatory milieu suggesting a "hot" tumor microenvironment, which is known to be more amenable to immune-based therapies, in particular checkpoint inhibitors. As such, the investigators found activation of cancer inflammatory gene sets in CDK12-mutant tumors (**Fig. 2**). More importantly, one patient who was treated with anti-PD-1 checkpoint inhibitor and had a PSA response following 4 cycles of drug, also had membranous and cytoplasmic staining of CD3 in addition to a radiographic response. As such, these results suggest that CDK12 may represent a potential biomarker in tumors with elevated neoantigen burden and that may benefit from checkpoint blockade. There are ongoing clinical trials in different clinical states: NCT04104893, a phase II study exploring activity and efficacy of pembrolizumab in veterans with mCRPC with either mismatch repair deficiency or CDK12 inactivation, and NCT03570619, a phase II trial using ipilimumab and nivolumab combination therapy followed by nivolumab monotherapy in patients with mCRPC harboring loss of CDK12 function, respectively, among others to further explore this hypothesis.

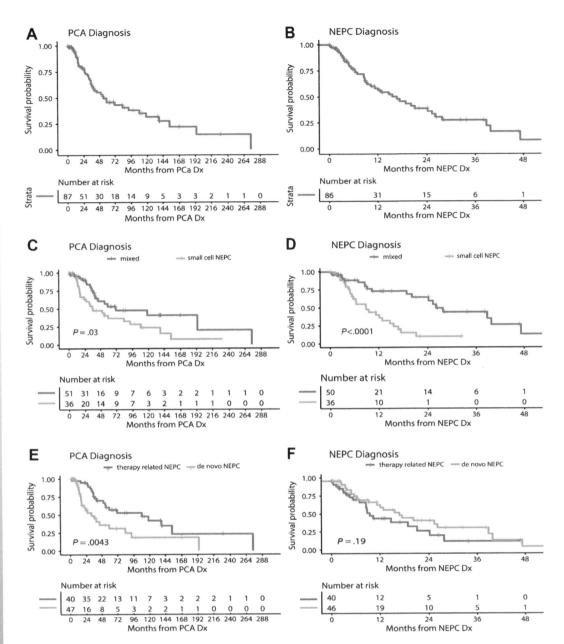

Fig. 1. OS in a cohort of patients with neuroendocrine prostate cancer showing multiple histologic patterns with neuroendocrine disease (NEPC). (*A*) OS from diagnoses of adenocarcinoma versus (*B*) diagnosis of NEPC. (*C*) OS of mixed histology. (*D*) Neuroendocrine histology. OS in de novo versus therapy-related NEPC from diagnosis of prostate cancer (*E*) and from diagnosis of NEPC (*F*). Different axes represent different time scales used for (*A*), (*C*), and (*E*) compared with (*B*), (*D*), and (*F*) due to different time intervals between OS from prostate cancer diagnosis and OS from NEPC diagnosis. (*From* Conteduca V, Oromendia C, Eng KW, et al. Clinical features of neuroendocrine prostate cancer. Eur J Cancer 2019; 121:7-18. doi:10.1016/j.ejca.2019.08.011; with permission.)

IMMUNOTHERAPY IN PRIME TIME: THE ROLE OF BIOMARKERS

A number of technology platforms are being implemented to assess peripheral blood and tissue based biomarkers; of these, RNA-sequencing, flow and mass cytometry, and enzyme-linked immunosorbent assay–based assays have been in widespread use.[24] There are still multiple challenges in using immune approaches in patients with mCRPC. It is clear that understanding the genetic background of the tumor and its host is

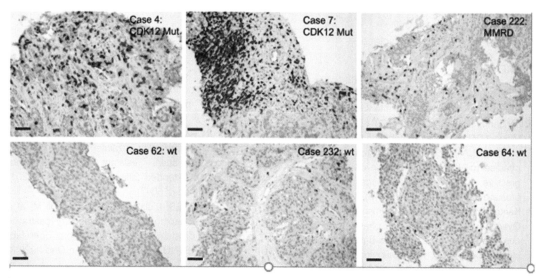

Fig. 2. Immunohistochemistry on formalin-fixed paraffin-embedded tumor sections showing T-cell infiltration by CD3+ cells. Six cases are shown, with 2 showcasing CDK12 mutant (Mut) tumors, 1 mismatch repair (MMR)-deficient tumor, and 3 that are wild type (wt) for CDK12, MMR genes, and homologous repair genes. (*From* Wu Y-M, Cieslik M, Lonigro RJ, et al. Inactivation of CDK12 delineates a distinct immunogenic class of advanced prostate cancer. Cell 2018; 173:1770-1782; with permission.)

highly relevant in certain cases, but at this time, one treatment does not fit all patients. Biomarkers may be in the form of changes in imaging using unique tracers, tumor mutational changes, mutational burden, presence or absence of programmed cell death (PD)-1 or PD-ligand 1 (PD-L1) on tumor or immune cells, circulating tumor cells, or tumor or cell-free DNA; however, biomarkers that are unique to assess changes within the tumor microenvironment or in the peripheral blood have not as yet been well-defined despite multiple efforts. Several solid tumors have relied on the presence of tumor-infiltrating lymphocytes (TILs) to develop and "immunoscore" to determine the amount of immunologic activity that is in situ within the tumor; however, prostate is unique in that it is rare to see TILs either at diagnosis or in the setting of progressive disease. The ratio of T regulatory cells (Tregs)/MDSCs has been explored; CD4+FOXP+CD24[hi] Tregs have been associated with poor prognosis. In addition, Treg frequency among TILs has been shown to correlate with tumor grade and reduced patient survival in several solid tumors, including breast, melanoma, glioblastoma, and ovarian cancers. What is now observed in multiple clinical trials with checkpoint inhibitors for several solid tumors, such as renal or urothelial cancers, is that the presence or absence of PD-L1 does not seem to impact treatment response. Gnjatic and colleagues[25] have provided guidance from Working Group 4 from the Society of Immunotherapy's Immune Biomarkers Task Force in an attempt to discover host genetic factors, tumor alterations in genes that affect APC function or affect local recruitment of inflammatory cells into the tumor microenvironment. Their work is one of many groups that continue to provide immune monitoring throughout the disease continuum in an effort to determine how to best characterize the immune system's role in disease response. These efforts are to be lauded, as they provide multidisciplinary, multi-institutional viewpoints that allow for greater insight into understanding the layers that govern the immune system's control of disease response.

DISCUSSION

There is a significant thrust toward the further genomic profiling of prostate tumors along the disease continuum, with each new clone likely harboring unique mutations to which novel drugs can be targeted. This does not, however, address the issue as to how to best target the disease in toto, as not all drugs target all sites of disease equally and sometimes not at all. We have come a very long way and are beginning to understand the conditions whereby the immune system can be better engaged with novel therapies. It is clear that no one drug is able to provide complete therapeutic response alone; therefore, continued efforts to combine different classes of agents along with immunologic therapies remain a viable long-term goal for researchers and practitioners alike.

DISCLOSURE

The author has nothing to disclose.

REFERENCES

1. Kantoff PW, Higano CS, Shore ND, et al. Sipuleucel-T immunotherapy for castration-resistant prostate cancer. N Engl J Med 2010;363:411–22.
2. McNeel DG, Eickhoff JC, Johnson LE, et al. Phase II trial of a DNA vaccine encoding Prostatic Acid Phosphatase (pTVG-HP [MVI-816] in patients with progressive, nonmetastatic, castration-sensitive prostate cancer. J Clin Onc 2019;37:3507–17.
3. Kantoff PW, Schuetz TJ, Blumentstein BA, et al. Overall survival analysis of a phase II randomized controlled trial of a poxviral-base PSA-targeted immunotherapy in metastatic castration-resistant prostate cancer. J Clin Onc 2010;28:1099–105.
4. Gulley JL, Borre M, Vogelzang NJ, et al. Phase III trial of PROSTVAC in asymptomatic or minimally symptomatic metastatic castration-resistant prostate cancer. J Clin Onc 2019;37:1051–61.
5. Gulley JL, Madan RA, Tsang Ky, et al. Immune impact induced by PROSTVAC (PSA-TRICOM), a therapeutic vaccine for prostate cancer. Cancer Immunol Res 2014;2:133–41.
6. Sek K, Molck C, Stewart GD, et al. Targeting adenosine receptor signaling in cancer therapy. Int J Mol Sci 2018;19:3837.
7. Vigano S, Alatzoglou D, Irving M, et al. Targeting adenosine in cancer immunotherapy to enhance T-cell function. Front Immunol 2019;10:925.
8. Mao W, Ghasemzadeh A, Freeman ZT, et al. Immunogenicity of prostate cancer is augmented by BET bromodomain inhibition. J Immunother Cancer 2019;7:277.
9. Slovin SF, Higano CS, Hamid O, et al. Ipilimumab alone or in combination with radiotherapy in metastatic castration-resistant prostate cancer: results from an open-label, multicenter phase I/II study. Ann Oncol 2013;24:1813–21.
10. Beer TM, Kwon ED, Drake CG, et al. Randomized, double-blind, phase III trial of Ipilimumab versus placebo in asymptomatic or minimally symptomatic patients with metastatic chemotherapy-naïve castration-resistant prostate cancer. J Clin Onc 2017;35:40–7.
11. Kwon ED, Drake CG, Scher HI, et al. Ipilimumab versus placebo after radiotherapy in patients with metastatic castration-resistant prostate cancer that had progressed after docetaxel chemotherapy CA184-043): a multicenter, randomised, double-blind, phase 3 trial. Lancet Oncol 2014;15:700–12.
12. Graff JN, Drake CG, Beer TM. Complete biochemical (Prostate-Specific Antigen) response to sipuleucel-T with enzalutamide in castration-resistant prostate cancer: A case report with implications for future research. Urology 2013;81:381–3.
13. Graff JN, Alumbal JJ, Drake CG, et al. Early evidence of anti-PD-1 activity in enzalutamide-resistant prostate cancer. Oncotarget 2016;7:52810–7.
14. Graff JN, Alumkal JJ, Thompson RF, et al. Pembrolizumab (Pembro) plus enzalutamide (Enz) in metastatic castration resistant prostate cancer (mCRPC): Extended followup. J Clin Oncol 2018;36 (suppl; abstr 5047).
15. Antonarakis ES, Piulats JM, Gross-Goupil M, et al. Pembrolizumab for treatment-refractory castration-resistant prostate cancer: multicohort, open-label phase II KEYNOTE-199 study. J Clin Onc 2020;38:395–405.
16. Slovin SF. Pembrolizumab in metastatic castration-resistant prostate cancer: Can an agnostic become a believer. J Clin Onc 2019;38:381–3.
17. Conteduca V, Oromendia C, Eng KW, et al. Clinical features of neuroendocrine prostate cancer. Eur J Cancer 2019;121:7–18.
18. Carreira S, Romanel A, Goodall J, et al. Tumor clone dynamics in lethal prostate cancer. Sci Transl Med 2014;6:254.
19. Aggarwal R, Huang J, Alumkal JI, et al. Clinical and genomic characterization of treatment-emergent small cell-neuroendocrine prostate cancer: a multi-institutional prospective study. J Clin Onc 2018;36:2492–503.
20. Akamatsu S, Wyatt AW, Lin D, et al. The placental gene PEG10 promotes progression of neuroendocrine prostate cancer. Cell Rep 2015;12:922–36.
21. Lin D, Dong X, Wang K, et al. Identification of DEK as a potential therapeutic target for neuroendocrine prostate cancer. Oncotarget 2015;6:1806–20.
22. Wu Y-M, Cieslik M, Lonigro RJ, et al. Inactivation of CDK12 delineates a distinct immunogenic class of advanced prostate cancer. Cell 2018;173:1770–82.
23. Cheng S-W, Kuzyk MA, Moradian A, et al. Interaction of cyclin-dependent kinase 12/CrkRS with cyclin K1 is required for the phosphorylation of the C-terminal domain of RNA polymerase II. Mol Cell Bio 2012;32:4691–704.
24. Nixon AB, Schalper KA, Jacobs I, et al. Peripheral immune-based biomarkers in cancer immunotherapy: can realize their predictive potential. J Immunother Cancer 2019;7:325.
25. Gnjatic S, Bronte V, Brunet LR, et al. Identifying baseline immune-related biomarkers to predict clinical outcome of immunotherapy. J Immunother Cancer 2017;5:44.

Application of Single-Cell Sequencing to Immunotherapy

Kristin G. Beaumont, PhD*, Michael A. Beaumont, PhD, Robert Sebra, PhD

KEYWORDS

- Immunotherapy • Cancer • Single-cell analysis • Prostate cancer • Urologic cancer
- Tumor heterogeneity

KEY POINTS

- Heterogeneity of a tumor and its microenvironment (including the immune compartment) likely contributes to differences in disease development and patient response to treatment.
- Next Generation Sequencing (NGS) of bulk tissue does not always capture heterogeneity.
- Single cell sequencing of cells from tissue allows for better resolution of minor cell populations.
- Understanding these populations can help identify tumor targets and cells that can be leveraged for immunotherapy as well as to understand the effects of therapy on tumor development.

INTRODUCTION

Cancer is a complex disease rooted in heterogeneity, which is the phenomenon of individual cells, tissues, or patients having distinct phenotypic and/or genetic characteristics. This is particularly true for cancers such as prostate cancer, in which the 200,000 new cases diagnosed each year are split between men diagnosed with clinically indolent disease that does not require immediate treatment and aggressive disease that requires intervention.[1] Similar heterogeneity is observed in therapeutic response, in which some patients relapse soon after treatment, but others remain disease free for years before recurring. Such divergent disease etiology is thought to be a result of tumor heterogeneity, and therefore, better understanding the complexity of this disease may inform better diagnosis and treatment.

Tumors evolve as cancerous cells grow within an intricate network of noncancerous cell types and extracellular matrix proteins, which taken together, comprise the tumor microenvironment (TME). It is only recently that the complexity of the TME has been appreciated for its role in cancer evolution, metastasis, and treatment outcomes, and that the varied subpopulations of cells (immune, stromal, cancer, and others) each uniquely contribute to the progression of disease. The classification of distinct and important subpopulations of cells within the tumor and its associated microenvironment has remained a technical challenge. Next generation sequencing (NGS) of bulk tumor tissue has yielded some exciting results, including the discovery of certain driver mutations and variants of unknown significance. In this approach, genetic material is extracted from bulk tissue and sequenced, which provides an overall average genetic profile of the sample, but masks contributions from individual cells and minor populations of cells, particularly in heterogeneous samples. Only with the advent of single-cell sequencing technologies has it become possible to characterize the key contributions of cell subpopulations to identify new therapeutic targets and disease biomarkers, and understand modes of treatment for disease, in which single-cell sequencing characterizes and reports the genome or transcriptome of each individual cell in a population, allowing the identification of subpopulations of

a Genetics and Genomic Sciences, Icahn School of Medicine at Mount Sinai, 1425 Madison Avenue, Box 1498, New York, NY 10029, USA
* Corresponding author.
E-mail address: kgbeaumont@gmail.com

Urol Clin N Am 47 (2020) 475–485
https://doi.org/10.1016/j.ucl.2020.07.005

cells that are genetically similar or distinct. This advantage is particularly important in characterizing and understanding tumor response to immunotherapy, as this therapeutic approach involves highly heterogeneous immune cell populations and tumor targets and bulk NGS approaches do not necessarily capture the complexity of such systems. In particular, single-cell analysis is uniquely suited to (1) identifying known, rare, or novel tumor targets; (2) characterizing patient-specific populations of immune cells that can be leveraged for immunotherapy; and (3) assessing the effects of immunotherapy on subpopulations of cells within a tumor to understand sensitivity or resistance. In this review, we view cancer immunotherapy through a single-cell lens and discuss the state-of-the art technologies that enable advances in this field.

HETEROGENEITY IN UROLOGIC CANCERS
Overview

Recognizing cancer as a highly heterogeneous disease is essential to studying its causes and evaluating therapeutic approaches. The extent of heterogeneity, which is the phenomenon of individual cells having distinct phenotypic and/or genomic/transcriptomic characteristics, is known to vary both as a function of disease and between patients with the same disease. For a given disease, heterogeneity may be defined as "interpatient" (mutational/transcriptional differences between tumors from different patients), "intrapatient" (mutational/transcriptional differences between tumors from the same patient, but derived from different sites), or "intratumor" (mutational/transcriptional differences between subpopulations within one tumor and its associated TME). Single-cell genomic and transcriptomic analyses facilitate a more comprehensive understanding of each level of heterogeneity, particularly intratumor heterogeneity (ITH), by permitting the identification and characterization of rare subpopulations of cells that were not previously detectable by bulk NGS methods. Moreover, single-cell analysis has been essential in identifying susceptible subpopulations of tumor cells that can serve as targets for immunotherapy, or identifying subsets of immune cells within the TME that can be leveraged for immunotherapy treatment (**Fig. 1**).

Heterogeneous tumors consist of many different cellular clones, or subpopulations of cells. The types and relative numbers of these cells differ between patients and tumors: there is now evidence that the degree of heterogeneity of a solid tumor and its associated TME affects its propensity to proliferate as well as its susceptibility to treatment. The clonal distribution of tumor cells may change during therapy, in an effect known as clonal evolution. Clonal evolution occurs when therapy targets only certain subsets of tumor cells, and the overall therapeutic profile of a tumor changes over the course of treatment: previously treatment-sensitive tumors may become treatment-

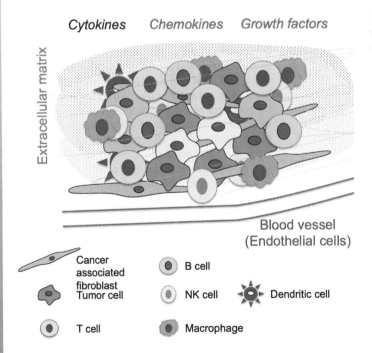

Fig. 1. Identifying subsets of immune cells within the TME that can be leveraged for immunotherapy treatment. NK cell, natural killer cell.

Cytokines   Chemokines   Growth factors

Extracellular matrix

Blood vessel (Endothelial cells)

Cancer associated fibroblast
Tumor cell
T cell
B cell
NK cell
Macrophage
Dendritic cell

resistant following therapy, where one possible consequence of therapy is preferential selection for survival of treatment-insensitive clones (which may be potentially rare and difficult to detect).[2] Leveraging single-cell data analysis to characterize clonal evolution following therapy can help inform clinicians as to the success of the approach or suggest whether a combined approach is necessary (**Fig. 2**).

As one particularly striking example, muscle invasive bladder cancer is known to have one of the highest mutation rates of any cancer, which results in extensive ITH at both the genomic and transcriptomic levels.[3] Although TP53 mutations were recognized early on as one of the key drivers of bladder cancer, targeting these tumors therapeutically yielded limited results, likely due at least in part to their highly heterogeneous nature. Cote and coworkers[4] authored an early report suggesting that patients bearing tumors with TP53 mutations responded better to chemotherapy, but follow-up clinical trials failed to support this observation. In one TP53-targeted phase III trial, which assessed treatment response to adjuvant cisplatin-based chemotherapy (vs surveillance)

based on TP53 status, yielded no difference in 5-year recurrence-free or overall survival based on this marker.[5] The investigators noted that immunohistochemistry, which was the primary method for assessing p53 dysregulation, likely failed to accurately reflect the range of patients' TP53 statuses, given that some mutations in TP53 result in p53 protein that is not reactive to the immunohistochemistry antibody.[6] This contradictory result was one of the first cautionary indicators that more detailed understanding of the characteristics of subpopulations of cells within these tumors was necessary to be able to predict therapeutic outcome.

Prostate cancer is also known to be particularly heterogeneous, starting even at the level of gross morphology. Classified as a "pluriform" neoplasm, it can consist of glandular, cribriform, trabecular, solid, and single-cell tumor patterns.[7] Moreover, prostate cancer is often multifocal, where some reports estimate that 50% to 90% of all radical prostatectomy specimens have more than one disease foci, and this characteristic is associated with higher grade, stage, and recurrence rates.[8] The origin of multifocal disease in prostate cancer is

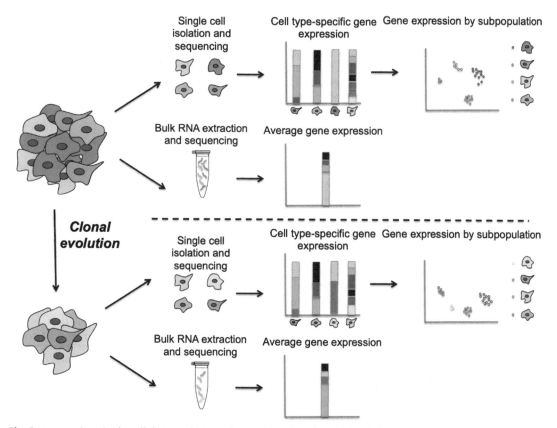

Fig. 2. Leveraging single-cell data analysis to characterize clonal evolution following therapy can help inform clinicians as to the success of the approach or suggest whether a combined approach is necessary.

not clear: one school of thought is that different genetic and epigenetic alterations occur in a single clone, which evolve through generations of daughter cells, resulting in different disease foci ("monoclonal origin"),[9] whereas an alternative view is that genetic abnormalities arise independently in otherwise healthy cells ("polyclonal origin," known as the cancer field effect).[10] Bulk sequencing of foci provides evidence supporting both views and clearly illustrates the genomic and transcriptomic heterogeneity in this disease.[11–14]

Heterogeneity in Immune Response

By definition, immunotherapy leverages the patient's own immune system to target tumor cells. The complexity of human immune response relies on the choreography of many different subpopulations of cells that are not only defined by cell type (eg, T cell, B cell, natural killer cell), but by state (activated, exhausted, cytotoxic). The necessity of single-cell analysis in characterizing immunotherapy mechanism and effectiveness becomes even more clear when heterogeneity in the immune response is considered alongside heterogeneity in the tumor and tumor-associated cells that will serve as targets for the immune campaign. Moreover, both sides of the immunotherapy coin (immune cells and their tumor targets) undergo phenotypic, genomic, and transcriptomic changes that vary spatially and temporally as well as in response to specific stimuli, further motivating the need for single-cell analysis of these effects.

Immune cells residing in the tumor microenvironment, or the tumor immune microenvironment (TIME), are particularly important in dictating tumor behavior and response to treatment. These populations of cells have been the focus of a great deal of recent research and are known to be highly heterogeneous in both identity and function. T cells and tumor-associated macrophages (TAMs) have both shown promise as biomarkers for immunotherapy, in which CD4+ helper T cells and cytotoxic CD8+ T cells can prevent tumor growth, and highly plastic TAMs can repress antitumor immunity, angiogenesis, and cell migration. In many cases, the makeup of the TIME can be used for predicting prognosis and is often associated with patient outcome. As one example, significant tumor infiltration of type 1 T-helper (Th1) cells, CD8+ cytotoxic T cells, and their associated cytokines typically suggest that a patient's immune system is capable of some degree of tumor suppression. Characterizing and defining an antitumor microenvironment is challenging given that tumor-associated immune cell populations vary by patient, disease subtype, and time. Furthermore, the function and interactions of different subpopulations have not been well-characterized, but studies toward this goal have yielded promising therapeutic targets, such as PD-1 and CTLA-4, which can be targeted by antibodies to overcome T-cell exhaustion.[15,16] Prostate cancer is somewhat unique in that it is both a known immunogenic disease and, for certain molecular subtypes, driven by hormone stimulation, making this an ideal disease for targeting with combination therapy. Designing combination therapy is inherently complex, particularly when both the tumor targets and immune system compartments are heterogeneous and temporally dynamic. It is also encouraging that prostate cancer has several well-described tumor-associated antigens (including prostate-specific antigen, prostatic acid phosphatase, and prostate-specific membrane antigen) that may serve as targets for immunotherapy.[17]

In evaluating immunotherapeutic approaches, single-cell analysis is uniquely suited to identifying tumor targets (known, rare, or novel), characterizing patient-specific populations of immune cells that can be leveraged for immunotherapy and assessing the effects of immunotherapy on subpopulations of cells within a tumor to understand sensitivity or resistance. One particularly notable example of using single-cell characterization to understand potential tumor response to immunotherapy was published by Chevrier and colleagues.[18] They developed an immune atlas of clear cell renal carcinoma from 73 affected patients and 5 healthy controls using single-cell mass cytometry (a complementary technique to single-cell sequencing that relies on antibody panels). By interrogating 3.5 million single cells, they identified 17 tumor-associated macrophage phenotypes and 22 T-cell phenotypes, but most significantly, were able to identify a signature immune composition that was associated with progression-free survival. This study clearly demonstrates that single-cell analysis reveals additional layers of cellular complexity and that this additional resolution can be clinically important.

Contributions of Bulk Next Generation Sequencing to Understanding Urologic Cancer

The Cancer Genome Atlas, the International Cancer Genome Consortium, and efforts of individual groups have illuminated some of the genetic roots of cancer (including prostate cancer) using bulk NGS approaches, such as whole genome sequencing (WGS), whole exome sequencing (WES), and bulk RNA sequencing.[19–24] These approaches rely on genetic material isolated from tissue and result in an average, overall genetic profile of the entire sample where the genetic contributions of individual cells are masked. Novel, common alterations have been identified in prostate cancer using this method, including SPOP and CHD1 mutations, and previously known targets have been validated (including PTEN and TP53 loss or mutation).[25] Using prostate cancer as a key example, though, the clinical utility of these efforts has been somewhat limited because, as one might expect, the genetics of this disease are very complex. Several genetic anomalies (fusions in ERG, ETV1/4, and FLI1 and mutations in SPOP, FOXa1, and IDH1) are common among patients with prostate cancer, and these have led to the evolution of 8 distinct molecular subtypes of the disease: 7 groups, each based on 1 conserved genetic alteration and 1 group of "other." However, samples within each of these classifications have demonstrated additional contributors to heterogeneity (for example, in epigenetic profiles and androgen-receptor activity) and these classifications have not been linked to either prognosis or therapeutic effectiveness.[7,19,26]

It is interesting that the Gleason score, which is a very strong predictor of disease progression in prostate cancer, has been demonstrated in some studies to be related to underlying genetic alterations.[7] As one example, Rubin and colleagues[27] performed WGS and WES on samples from 426 prostate cancer samples, with the goal of identifying genomic support for prognostic grade groupings, which are clinical categorizations based on Gleason number. They observed increasing polyploidal frequency with increases in genomic amplification, deletions, and nonsynonymous point mutations with increasing grade.[27] This observation, taken together with the knowledge that single-cell analysis can better characterize the genetic complexity of disease, leads to the hope that single-cell sequencing and characterization may contribute significantly toward clinically actionable information, particularly in highly heterogeneous treatment scenarios, such as immunotherapy of urologic cancers.

Single-Cell Sequencing: Current State of the Art

Single-cell sequencing has grown extensively in the past several years, both in the characterization of single-cell genomics (DNA) and single-cell transcriptomics (RNA). Single-cell genomic analysis has been particularly useful in understanding the evolution of somatic mutations in disease. As one example, Zhang and coworkers[28] used single-cell WGS to characterize the somatic mutational landscape in B lymphocytes as a function of age and found that cells from newborns contained fewer than 500 mutations per cell, whereas cells from centenarians contained more than 3000 mutations per cell. They were also able to use this approach to identify mutational hotspot regions, some of which were located at genes associated with somatic hypermutations, similar to mutational signatures observed in B-cell tumors.[28]

Single-cell transcriptomic analysis reflects the functional diversity of cells and can capture the functional consequences of tumor/TME interactions as well as the effects of treatment. As one cogent example, Horning and coworkers[29] used single-cell RNA sequencing to characterize prostate cancer cell response to androgen stimulation, given that there is evidence that small androgen-independent subclones of cells are preferentially selected during androgen deprivation therapy and drive post-therapy disease progression. In this work, they profiled the transcriptomes of 144 single LNCaP prostate cancer cells, following cell-cycle synchronization and androgen treatment, which revealed previously unappreciated heterogeneity in the cellular response of 8 potential subpopulations. In particular, they identified one subpopulation of cells with enhanced expression of 10 cell-cycle genes, and decreased dependence on androgen-receptor signaling, which resulted in advanced growth and sphere formation capability of these cells. This work clearly highlights the need to understand the heterogeneity in this disease to better understand disease progression and therapeutic mechanism.

Single-cell immune profiling approaches also have proven useful in understanding immune response at the single-cell level. In brief, the V(D)J sequences of T cells and B cells are characterized such that T-cell and B-cell clonotype diversity profiles and antigen specificity can be evaluated. This is invaluable not only as an additional dimension for understanding the TIME, but also in evaluating personalized medicine approaches.

OVERVIEW OF SINGLE-CELL SEQUENCING APPROACHES
Single-Cell DNA Sequencing

Although much of the discussion in this review has been focused on the value of single-cell transcriptomics (via single-cell RNA sequencing), it is important to note that single-cell characterization of the genome has also been evolving toward novel and impactful data (**Fig. 3**). Single-cell copy number variation analysis has proven useful

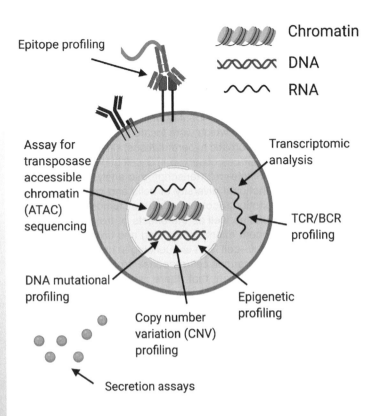

Fig. 3. Single-cell characterization of the genome has also been evolving toward novel and impactful data.

in characterizing genomic heterogeneity and clonal evolution, particularly in diseases driven by such aberrations (such as multiple myeloma).[30] Single-cell approaches to understanding epigenetic heterogeneity have also been developed, particularly those aimed at characterizing chromatin accessibility (single-cell assay for transposase-accessible chromatin sequencing)[31,32] and methylation,[33] where these data are useful in understanding accessibility and activity of transcriptional promoters.

Single-Cell RNA Sequencing

Early, plate-based approaches to single-cell analysis focused on single-cell isolation followed by Smart-Seq library preparation and Illumina-based sequencing. There are a variety of methods that have been useful for single-cell isolation, including laser dissection, targeted fluorescence-activated cell sorting (FACS), or more novel microfluidic approaches such as the C1 (Fluidigm, South San Francisco, CA), DEPArray (Menarini Silicon Biosystems, Bologna, Italy), or Beacon (Berkeley Lights, Emeryville, CA). Cells are directly sorted into well plates containing cell lysis buffer and reagents for reverse transcription. The resulting complementary DNA (cDNA) then undergoes amplification and tagmentation in preparation for

short-read NGS sequencing, where libraries are prepared cell by cell and then barcoded before pooling. Although these methods are highly useful in that they yield full-length transcripts for each cell, throughput is limited by sorting capacity, manual effort required for library preparation, and per cell cost.

Droplet-Based Single-Cell RNA Sequencing Approaches

To address the limited throughput of plate-based approaches, several groups have developed droplet-based approaches (Drop-Seq and InDrop); these are the most recent innovative approaches that facilitate the isolation and sequencing of large numbers (thousands) of single cells in a highly efficient manner.[34,35] Droplet-based methods combine single-cell isolation (via Poisson loading of single cells into fluid droplets) with cell lysis; in this approach, single cells in suspension flow into a microfluidic network and are captured into fluid droplets that also contain all the necessary reagents for cell lysis, messenger RNA (mRNA) capture/labeling with a Unique Molecular Identifier (UMI), and reverse transcription. Then, cDNA is amplified and libraries are constructed for short-read NGS sequencing, where droplet (and usually single-cell) identity is retained by a barcode. Sequencing is initiated from either the 3′ or 5′ end of the transcript, but current read lengths (100–150 base pairs) yield only partial information from the transcript. Research efforts demonstrating targeted, long-read/full-length, single-cell sequencing (ie, scIsoSeq) are ongoing and aim to address this current limitation.[36]

TECHNICAL CONSIDERATIONS IN SINGLE-CELL SEQUENCING
Sample Preparation and Handling

One of the major challenges associated with any approach to single-cell sequencing is in the generation and/or selection of single viable, intact cells from tissue; this is particularly true as more and more patient and patient-derived samples are being interrogated via this method.[37] Tumor or tissue dissociation requires optimization and validation to ensure that all populations are appropriately represented and that disaggregation methods do not selectively lyse sensitive cells. Moreover, enrichment for cell populations of interest is often necessary and strategies to accomplish this (eg, depletion of bulk cells, targeted FACS, bead-based enrichment of target cells) must also be optimized and validated. Dynamic changes in the tissue and isolated cells also must be considered in designing and evaluating single-cell experiments; changes in cell health, signaling, and transcription (even those induced solely from dissociation) will all be reflected in single-cell sequencing data, particularly as the sensitivity of this method increases.

Number of Cells Analyzed and Sequencing Depth

One important consideration in designing single-cell analyses is the size of the cell population of interest; this is especially true if rare cell populations are the target of a study, as many fold more total cells must be analyzed to yield information from a sufficient number of rare cells (where, for example, rare cells might be treatment-resistant clones, circulating tumor cells, or cancer stem cells) with adequate sequencing depth (historically 50,000–100,000 reads per cell for differential gene expression analysis, where deeper sequencing can reveal additional genes up to the point of sequencing saturation).[37] This is a very important clinical consideration when analyzing samples from patients who are either at an early stage of their disease or have low levels of refractory disease, as cells of interest from these patients may be present in very low numbers. In some cases, it is necessary to combine cells derived from multiple samples/patients/animals to achieve the total

number of cells required; this is especially true when analyzing small tumor biopsies or highly acellular tissue (such as some bladder tumors). Although retaining the sample identity of single cells is straightforward in plate-based approaches, historically, this has been more challenging for droplet-based methods, as there is no way to track droplets through the microfluidic system. Recent advances, such as "cell hashing," enable the pooling, analysis and de-multiplexing of multiple samples such that data from individual cells can be traced back to their original sample source.[38] In this novel approach, oligonucleotide barcoded antibodies (or "hashtags") that ubiquitously recognize cell membrane proteins are used to label individual cell populations before pooling, where each sample is labeled with a different oligonucleotide sequence and the hashtag oligonucleotides are sequenced alongside the cDNA libraries to permit sample assignment of each cell.

Scale

Handling samples on a cell-by-cell basis from isolation to sequencing can be prohibitively cumbersome and labor-intensive, so a number of approaches have been developed that permit multiplexing of cells to increase the efficiency of this process. Incorporation of cell barcoding allows mRNA from many cells to be sequenced in one batch, where de-multiplexing can be performed computationally in the analysis phase; the approach has been incorporated into single-cell sequencing methods such as single-cell RNA barcoding and sequencing (SCRB-Seq),[39] massively parallel single-cell RNA sequencing (MARS-Seq),[40] and cell expression by linear amplification sequencing (Cel-Seq).[41] Furthermore, as described previously, the addition of microfluidics has increased the handling efficiency, and capacity of several techniques. Although conceptually Drop-seq relies on microfluidics to enable droplet loading, companies such as 10X Genomics (Pleasanton, CA), BioRad (Hercules, CA), and Fluidigm have engineered platforms that combine microfluidic devices and cell barcoding to enable cDNA generation from hundreds to thousands of single cells at once.

Data Handling/Analysis

As single-cell sequencing data becomes more cost-effective, the shift from molecular and biologic bottlenecks to data handling is apparent. For example, single-cell RNA sequencing typically targets 50,000 to 100,000 transcript reads per cell to enable differential expression analysis.

Transcripts are counted by the addition of UMIs and aligned against a reference for gene calling. Most commonly, data are filtered to remove background (too few UMIs), unhealthy/dead cells (as determined by the percentage of mitochondrial reads from a given cells), and doublets/multiplets. Data normalization is then performed by scaling count data to correct relative gene abundances between cells, followed by correction methods (to remove effects of technical batch or cell-cycle variation). Given that up to approximately 25,000 genes are part of the original single-cell data set, it becomes necessary to reduce the analysis to genes that are most interesting, and are most variable between cells, which is done by feature selection to reduce the dimensionality of the dataset to the most interesting approximately 500 to 5000 genes. Further dimensionality reduction is done using principal component analysis and a nonlinear reduction method, such as t-SNE,[42] or uniform manifold approximation and projection (UMAP)[43] to facilitate cluster visualization. The resulting clusters are then annotated based on genes expressed, both for identity (ie, clusters with high CD4 expression are T cells) and, to some extent, for function (ie, clusters with high granzyme B and lysozyme are likely cytotoxic). Additional downstream analyses, such as trajectory analysis, in which clusters are related to each other sequentially by differential gene expression profile, are also becoming more common.[44] Also, machine learning approaches have been leveraged to dig deeper into large (typically bulk) sequencing data sets to try to find correlations between clinical metrics and gene expression.[45,46]

There are still many challenges associated with single-cell RNA sequencing data analysis. With increasing experimental throughput, single-cell datasets have become prohibitively large for the average personal computer. Access to high-performance computing options has become a necessity in many cases. Data analysis methods have exploded in parallel with single-cell experimental approaches, and it has become important for investigators to optimize and select the most appropriate filtering, normalization and dimensionality reduction strategies for their data sets. Finally, annotation of clusters by gene expression is still largely manual in many cases, which presents challenges in both bandwidth and consistency.

EMERGING TECHNOLOGIES
Other –Omics

As single-cell sequencing technologies develop, investigators have had the opportunity to ask increasingly challenging research questions that require integration of complex cellular phenotype data with sequencing data. Approaches, such as cellular indexing of transcriptomes and epitopes by sequencing (CITE-seq), where markers for cellular protein expression are combined with Drop-seq–based cell isolation and processing, have begun to address these challenges, allowing sequencing information to be linked to characterized cells.[47] However, the types of phenotypic data that can be linked to sequencing data are currently limited to surface protein expression that can be labeled with an antibody. Other types of characteristic phenotypic data, such as growth kinetics, secretion, or cellular function, are not accessible by these methods, and require more sophisticated approaches.[48]

Single-Cell Multi-Omic Integration

Active efforts are under way to enable integration of data from multiple single-cell analytical methods, including single-cell DNA and RNA sequencing, with single-cell proteomics. Such multilayered analysis will provide the most complete characterization of the tumor and its associated microenvironment, both during the development of disease and in response to therapy. Some of the most exciting examples of these approaches include CITE-Seq (described previously, which pairs single-cell RNA sequencing and surface protein analysis),[47] Genotyping of Transcriptomes, or GoT (which pairs DNA sequencing and RNA sequencing for the same cell),[49] and combining single-cell DNA methylation analysis with RNA sequencing.[50]

Spatial Sequencing

One very significant caveat to single-cell sequencing is that it requires isolated cells that, by definition, have been removed from their anatomic context. Given the increasing appreciation for spatial and temporal heterogeneity as well as the role of dynamic cellular interactions in disease progression, it has become critical to develop methods that retain the spatial context of individual cells. To this end, several spatial sequencing approaches (such as Slide-Seq,[51] multiplexed error-robust fluorescence in situ hybridization [MERFISH],[52] spatially resolved transcript amplicon readout mapping [STARmap][53] and the Visium assay from 10X Genomics) have been developed and are now approaching single-cell resolution. The methods are similar to single-cell transcriptomic approaches, but are used on a slide-mounted intact sample (such as a tissue slice) and leverage a spatial barcode that allows the registration of transcripts to their position on the slide.

This novel approach was used to characterize spatially resolved gene expression in 6750 tissue regions within a Gs 3 + 4 adenocarcinoma prostate tumor section. Berglund and colleagues[54] were able to resolve extensive intratumor heterogeneity and identify distinct expression profiles for tissue compartments, including normal, cancer, stroma, immune cell, and prostatic intraepithelial neoplasia glands. Moreover, they were able to resolve the high degree of inflammation and immune response in tumor and adjacent normal tissue, compared with normal tissue. In short, this approach (particularly when combined with large-scale analysis of matched single cells) will add spatial complexity and dimensionality to single-cell sequencing and even further increase the promise of this method.

SUMMARY

Cancer is a highly complex and heterogeneous disease, and immunotherapy has shown promise as a therapeutic approach. Although bulk NGS has helped to broadly inform treatment of cancer (including with immunotherapy), the increased resolution afforded by single-cell analysis offers the hope of finding and characterizing previously underappreciated populations of cells that could prove useful in understanding the progression and treatment of cancer. In evaluating immunotherapeutic approaches, single-cell analysis is uniquely suited to (1) identifying known, rare, or novel tumor targets; (2) characterizing patient-specific populations of immune cells that can be leveraged for immunotherapy; and (3) assessing the effects of immunotherapy on subpopulations of cells within a tumor to understand sensitivity or resistance. Urologic and prostate cancers are inherently heterogeneous diseases, even as far as cancer is concerned, and the potential for single-cell analysis to help understand and develop immunotherapeutic approaches to treat these diseases is very exciting. Further advances in these technologies to interweave multiple –omics methods with spatial analysis of the tumor immune microenvironment promises to bring our understanding of the evolution of cancer and effects of immunotherapy to an entirely new level, which will hopefully translate to great improvement in clinical outcomes.

CLINICAL COMMENTS

- Heterogeneity of a tumor and its microenvironment (including the immune compartment)

likely contributes to differences in disease development and patient response to treatment.
- NGS of bulk tissue does not always capture heterogeneity.
- Single-cell sequencing of cells from tissue allows for better resolution of different minor cell populations, which can help identify tumor targets, identify cells that can be leveraged for immunotherapy, and to understand the effects of therapy on tumor development.

DISCLOSURE

The authors declare no commercial or financial conflicts of interest.

REFERENCES

1. Yadav SS, Stockert JA, Hackert V, et al. Intratumor heterogeneity in prostate cancer. Urol Oncol 2018; 36(8):349–60.
2. Riaz N, Havel JJ, Makarov V, et al. Tumor and Microenvironment Evolution during Immunotherapy with Nivolumab. Cell 2017;171(4):934–49.e16.
3. da Costa JB, Gibb EA, Nykopp TK, et al. Molecular tumor heterogeneity in muscle invasive bladder cancer: Biomarkers, subtypes, and implications for therapy. Urol Oncol 2018. https://doi.org/10.1016/j.urolonc.2018.11.015.
4. Cote RJ, Esrig D, Groshen S, et al. p53 and treatment of bladder cancer. Nature 1997;385(6612): 123–5.
5. Stadler WM, Lerner SP, Groshen S, et al. Phase III study of molecularly targeted adjuvant therapy in locally advanced urothelial cancer of the bladder based on p53 status. J Clin Oncol 2011;29(25): 3443–9.
6. George B, Datar RH, Wu L, et al. p53 gene and protein status: the role of p53 alterations in predicting outcome in patients with bladder cancer. J Clin Oncol 2007;25(34):5352–8.
7. Tolkach Y, Kristiansen G. The heterogeneity of prostate cancer: a practical approach. Pathobiology 2018;85(1-2):108–16.
8. Djavan B, Susani M, Bursa B, et al. Predictability and significance of multifocal prostate cancer in the radical prostatectomy specimen. Tech Urol 1999; 5(3):139–42.
9. Trujillo KA, Jones AC, Griffith JK, et al. Markers of field cancerization: proposed clinical applications in prostate biopsies. Prostate Cancer 2012;2012: 302894.
10. Slaughter DP, Southwick HW, Smejkal W. Field cancerization in oral stratified squamous epithelium; clinical implications of multicentric origin. Cancer 1953;6(5):963–8.

11. Andreoiu M, Cheng L. Multifocal prostate cancer: biologic, prognostic, and therapeutic implications. Hum Pathol 2010;41(6):781–93.

12. Boyd LK, Mao X, Xue L, et al. High-resolution genome-wide copy-number analysis suggests a monoclonal origin of multifocal prostate cancer. Genes Chromosomes Cancer 2012;51(6):579–89.

13. Kobayashi M, Ishida H, Shindo T, et al. Molecular analysis of multifocal prostate cancer by comparative genomic hybridization. Prostate 2008;68(16):1715–24.

14. Lindberg J, Klevebring D, Liu W, et al. Exome sequencing of prostate cancer supports the hypothesis of independent tumour origins. Eur Urol 2013;63(2):347–53.

15. Ribas A. Releasing the brakes on cancer immunotherapy. N Engl J Med 2015;373(16):1490–2.

16. Shin DS, Ribas A. The evolution of checkpoint blockade as a cancer therapy: what's here, what's next? Curr Opin Immunol 2015;33:23–35.

17. Schepisi G, Farolfi A, Conteduca V, et al. Immunotherapy for prostate cancer: where we are headed. Int J Mol Sci 2017;18(12).

18. Chevrier S, Levine JH, Zanotelli VRT, et al. An immune atlas of clear cell renal cell carcinoma. Cell 2017;169(4):736–49.e18.

19. The molecular taxonomy of primary prostate cancer. Cell 2015;163(4):1011–25.

20. Barbieri CE, Baca SC, Lawrence MS, et al. Exome sequencing identifies recurrent SPOP, FOXA1 and MED12 mutations in prostate cancer. Nat Genet 2012;44(6):685–9.

21. Blattner M, Lee DJ, O'Reilly C, et al. SPOP mutations in prostate cancer across demographically diverse patient cohorts. Neoplasia 2014;16(1):14–20.

22. Grisanzio C, Werner L, Takeda D, et al. Genetic and functional analyses implicate the NUDT11, HNF1B, and SLC22A3 genes in prostate cancer pathogenesis. Proc Natl Acad Sci U S A 2012;109(28):11252–7.

23. Pflueger D, Rickman DS, Sboner A, et al. N-myc downstream regulated gene 1 (NDRG1) is fused to ERG in prostate cancer. Neoplasia 2009;11(8):804–11.

24. Pflueger D, Terry S, Sboner A, et al. Discovery of non-ETS gene fusions in human prostate cancer using next-generation RNA sequencing. Genome Res 2011;21(1):56–67.

25. Yadav SS, Li J, Lavery HJ, et al. Next-generation sequencing technology in prostate cancer diagnosis, prognosis, and personalized treatment. Urol Oncol 2015;33(6):267.e1-13.

26. Mian OY, Tendulkar RD, Abazeed ME. The evolving role of molecular profiling in prostate cancer: basal and luminal subtyping transcends tissue of origin. Transl Cancer Res 2017;6(Suppl 9):S1441–5.

27. Rubin MA, Girelli G, Demichelis F. Genomic correlates to the newly proposed grading prognostic groups for prostate cancer. Eur Urol 2016;69(4):557–60.

28. Zhang L, Dong X, Lee M, et al. Single-cell whole-genome sequencing reveals the functional landscape of somatic mutations in B lymphocytes across the human lifespan. Proc Natl Acad Sci U S A 2019;116(18):9014–9.

29. Horning AM, Wang Y, Lin CK, et al. Single-cell RNA-seq reveals a subpopulation of prostate cancer cells with enhanced cell-cycle-related transcription and attenuated androgen response. Cancer Res 2018;78(4):853–64.

30. Prideaux SM, Conway O'Brien E, Chevassut TJ. The genetic architecture of multiple myeloma. Adv Hematol 2014;2014:864058.

31. Buenrostro JD, Wu B, Chang HY, et al. ATAC-seq: a method for assaying chromatin accessibility genome-wide. Curr Protoc Mol Biol 2015;109:21.29.1–21.29.9.

32. Buenrostro JD, Wu B, Litzenburger UM, et al. Single-cell chromatin accessibility reveals principles of regulatory variation. Nature 2015;523(7561):486–90.

33. Smallwood SA, Lee HJ, Angermueller C, et al. Single-cell genome-wide bisulfite sequencing for assessing epigenetic heterogeneity. Nat Methods 2014;11(8):817–20.

34. Klein AM, Mazutis L, Akartuna I, et al. Droplet barcoding for single-cell transcriptomics applied to embryonic stem cells. Cell 2015;161(5):1187–201.

35. Macosko EZ, Basu A, Satija R, et al. Highly parallel genome-wide expression profiling of individual cells using nanoliter droplets. Cell 2015;161(5):1202–14.

36. Gupta I, Collier PG, Haase B, et al. Single-cell isoform RNA sequencing characterizes isoforms in thousands of cerebellar cells. Nat Biotechnol 2018. https://doi.org/10.1038/nbt.4259.

37. Kolodziejczyk AA, Kim JK, Svensson V, et al. The technology and biology of single-cell RNA sequencing. Mol Cell 2015;58(4):610–20.

38. Stoeckius M, Zheng S, Houck-Loomis B, et al. Cell hashing with barcoded antibodies enables multiplexing and doublet detection for single cell genomics. Genome Biol 2018;19(1):224.

39. Soumillon M, Cacchiarelli D, Semrau S, et al. Characterization of directed differentiation by high-throughput single-cell RNA-Seq. BioRxiv 2014. https://doi.org/10.1101/003236.

40. Jaitin DA, Kenigsberg E, Keren-Shaul H, et al. Massively parallel single-cell RNA-seq for marker-free decomposition of tissues into cell types. Science 2014;343(6172):776–9.

41. Ziegenhain C, Vieth B, Parekh S, et al. Comparative analysis of single-cell RNA sequencing methods. Mol Cell 2017;65(4):631–43.e4.

42. van der Maaten L, Hinton G. Visualizing data using t-SNE. Journal of Machine Learning Research 2008;9: 2579–605.

43. Becht E, McInnes L, Healy J, et al. Dimensionality reduction for visualizing single-cell data using UMAP. Nat Biotechnol 2018. https://doi.org/10.1038/nbt.4314.

44. Qiu X, Mao Q, Tang Y, et al. Reversed graph embedding resolves complex single-cell trajectories. Nat Methods 2017;14(10):979–82.

45. Glaab E, Bacardit J, Garibaldi JM, et al. Using rule-based machine learning for candidate disease gene prioritization and sample classification of cancer gene expression data. PLoS One 2012;7(7):e39932.

46. Singh D, Febbo PG, Ross K, et al. Gene expression correlates of clinical prostate cancer behavior. Cancer Cell 2002;1(2):203–9.

47. Stoeckius M, Hafemeister C, Stephenson W, et al. Simultaneous epitope and transcriptome measurement in single cells. Nat Methods 2017;14(9):865–8.

48. Beaumont KG, Hamou W, Bozinovic N, et al. Multi-parameter cell characterization using nanofluidic technology facilitates real-time phenotypic and genotypic elucidation of intratumor heterogeneity. bioRxiv 2018. https://doi.org/10.1101/457010.

49. Nam AS, Kim KT, Chaligne R, et al. Somatic mutations and cell identity linked by genotyping of transcriptomes. Nature 2019;571(7765):355–60.

50. Zhou F, Wang R, Yuan P, et al. Reconstituting the transcriptome and DNA methylome landscapes of human implantation. Nature 2019;572(7771):660–4.

51. Rodriques SG, Stickels RR, Goeva A, et al. Slide-seq: a scalable technology for measuring genome-wide expression at high spatial resolution. Science 2019;363(6434):1463–7.

52. Xia C, Babcock HP, Moffitt JR, et al. Multiplexed detection of RNA using MERFISH and branched DNA amplification. Sci Rep 2019;9(1):7721.

53. Wang X, Allen WE, Wright MA, et al. Three-dimensional intact-tissue sequencing of single-cell transcriptional states. Science 2018;361(6400).

54. Berglund E, Maaskola J, Schultz N, et al. Spatial maps of prostate cancer transcriptomes reveal an unexplored landscape of heterogeneity. Nat Commun 2018;9(1):2419.

Immunotherapy for Metastatic Prostate Cancer: Current and Emerging Treatment Options

Dimple Chakravarty, DVM, PhD[a],*, Li Huang, MD, PhD[b,c],
Matthew Kahn, MS[b], Ashutosh K. Tewari, MD[a]

KEYWORDS

- Prostate cancer • Immunotherapy • Vaccines • Checkpoint inhibition therapy • Preclinical models

KEY POINTS

- The advent of immunotherapy has revolutionized treatment for patients with cancer.
- Recent studies have reported that, despite low mutation burden, prostate cancer has a high number of DNA damage and repair gene defects that makes prostate cancer immune sensitive.
- Immunotherapies that have been tested in prostate cancer so far have been mainly vaccines and checkpoint inhibitors.
- What holds promise is a combination of genomically targeted therapies (gene and cell therapies), with approaches to alleviate immune response and thereby make the tumor microenvironment immunologically "hot."

PROGRESSION

Cancer is a disease of major concern worldwide and is the second leading cause of mortality.[1] The United States remains one of the countries with the highest incidence rates of prostate cancer.[2] Histologically, 93% of prostate cancer occurs as acinar adenocarcinoma. The remaining 7% of the prostate cancers are variations of ductal adenocarcinoma, basal cell carcinoma, and neuroendocrine tumors. The latter cancer forms are not as common as the acinar adenocarcinoma in the preliminary stages of prostate cancer. It is also difficult to distinguish between acinar adenocarcinoma and intraductal carcinoma because they frequently present together.[3] However, through the progression of drug treatments and different therapeutic regimes for patients with prostate cancer, neuroendocrine tumors can appear in much as 20% in patient populations with castration-resistant prostate cancer (CRPC).[4–7]

Like other tumor types, the occurrence and subsequent development of prostate cancer seem to be driven by genetic aberrations, mutations, and variations. Specifically, the genetic alterations found to be associated with primary prostate cancer include ERG, ETV1, ETV4, FLI1, SPOP, FOXA1, and IDH1.[8] To understand the complexity of prostate cancer is to not only recognize the differences between tumors in patients, but also the heterogeneity between the tumor cells within the patient. In this case, the molecular heterogeneity is grounded in differences from genes to transcriptomic expression. There is not one determinant of tumor development and pathogenesis.[9] TMPRSS2-ERG fusion is seen is approximately 40% to 50% of patients diagnosed with prostate cancer,[10,11] whereas SPOP missense mutations are present in 6% to 15% of cases.[12] TMPRSS2-ERG fusion results from the fusion of these 2 genes on 2 different chromosomes. The result of

a Department of Urology and the Tisch Cancer Institute, Icahn School of Medicine at Mount Sinai, New York, NY 10029, USA; b Department of Urology, Icahn School of Medicine at Mount Sinai, New York, New York, USA; c Department of Urology, Sun Yat-sen Memorial Hospital, Sun Yat-sen University, Guangzhou, China
* Corresponding author.
E-mail address: dimple.chakravarty@mountsinai.org

Urol Clin N Am 47 (2020) 487–510
https://doi.org/10.1016/j.ucl.2020.07.010
0094-0143/20/© 2020 Elsevier Inc. All rights reserved.

this fusion is the enhancement of androgen dependency and the development of cancer.[11,13] Despite occurring in such a high fraction of the patients with prostate cancer, it does not seem to be a good prognosticator.[14] SPOP mutations are seen to be present in both localized and metastatic prostate cancers.[12] It has been shown to be involved in the ubiquitination of proteins and possibly has a role in maintaining genomic stability.[15] Another important genetic alteration associated with prostate cancer is the genomic deletion of PTEN gene.[8,16] PTEN deletion is seen in 40% to 60% of patients with prostate cancer[8,17] and it functions by inhibiting the PI3K/Akt signaling and inducing cell cycle arrest.[18]

Specific tumor suppressor proteins like Rb1 and Trp53 assist in the maintenance of the cell cycle by halting aberrant growth. Genomic alterations in TP53 involve mostly loss of function mutations or homozygous deletion and it is evidenced in 40% to 60% of prostate cancer cases, predominantly in metastatic prostate cancer.[8,19] Their relation to prostate cancer is important because the inhibition of the genes coding for Rb1 and Trp53 facilitates the cancer's ability to develop androgen deprivation therapy resistance thus paving the way for metastatic development. It was shown that the loss of both Rb1 and Trp53 in mice led to a significant decrease in survival after several weeks compared with single knockout mice groups. Thus, their loss controls linear plasticity in cancer cells in the sense that mutation can eventually lead to insensitivity to drug therapy.[20] Furthermore, SOX2 expression is significantly amplified with double loss of Trp53 and Rb1, indicating that its elevation is correlated with these other genes in controlling cancer.[21]

Primary prostate cancer or early stage prostate cancer is a very localized disease with limited growth. Accompanying this stage are low prostate-specific antigen (PSA) levels and Gleason scores, compared with later metastasis and more severe cases of prostate cancer. If identified at an early stage, several treatment options are available to the patient, such as active surveillance, radiation therapy, and even radical prostatectomy.[22] Active surveillance involves monitoring blood PSA levels or using digital rectal examinations. Radiation therapy is a technique that uses a high beam of radiation to kill dividing cancer cells. Radical prostatectomy is another standard procedure for removing the entire prostate organ and has shown significant efficacy in decreasing cancer development.[22] Patients can be divided into different groups depending on the characteristics of primary prostate cancer, such as low-, intermediate-, and high-risk groups.

Prostate cancer progresses from localized forms in the prostate gland, spreading to surrounding tissues, and subsequently metastasizing to distant sites like the vertebral bone. As the cancer cells grow and mutate, there are changes in the biochemical and pathologic development of the tumor microenvironment that can be controlled by various drug treatments and therapeutic regimes. When a patient has advanced prostate cancer, androgen deprivation therapy is recommended because the cancer cells rely heavily on androgen receptor signaling. These androgen receptors respond to testosterone and dihydrotestosterone for effective signaling and cell growth. Luteinizing hormone-releasing hormone (LHRH) antagonists are useful drugs in this case because they inhibit the production of the luteinizing hormone and prevent the synthesis of testosterone in the testes. These drug therapies are usually administered when the primary prostate cancer is ADT sensitive.

In the castrate-sensitive phase, local therapies include external beam radiation and implant radiation, high-intensity ultrasound therapy, surgeries such as radical prostatectomy and orchiectomy (very uncommon owing to psychological implications), and androgen deprivation therapy in the form of LHRH analogs that interfere with normal hormonal balances by diminishing the production of testosterone and thus dihydrotestosterone. However, cancer can become resistant to the hormonal drug therapies and become insensitive to androgen deprivation therapy. This specific form is known as CRPC. Treatments for castrate-resistant disease include combinations of abiraterone and prednisolone/enzalutamide, as well as docetaxel.

The discussion of drug therapies elsewhere in this article represents the common protocol in the treatment of prostate cancer. However, novel drugs and phase I trial combination therapies are continually being researched. It is important to think about the medical interventions and potential areas for targeted therapy that can obstruct and inhibit cancer survival.

The purpose of external beam radiation therapy is to ablate the prostate tumor using an external source of high energy. Tomita and colleagues[23] looked at the effect of high-intensity radiation on clinical relapse along with neoadjuvant androgen deprivation therapy and found significant improvements for intermediate as well as high-risk patients with prostate cancer. Other studies from Preisser and colleagues[24] discovered that external beam radiation in patients who underwent previous radical prostatectomy showed different patterns in terms of surrounding tissue toxicity. Tissue toxicity is an important factor in deciding whether or not to use certain treatment options and age differences should be taken into account. What they found was that secondary primary cancers resulting from external beam radiation–induced bladder cancer as the second most common site outranking skin cancer.[24] Furthermore, another study sought to understand changes in PSA levels resulting from the use of implant radiation. D'Amico and colleagues[25] found that implant radiation combined with neoadjuvant androgen deprivation therapy had significantly reduced PSA levels compared with just radical prostatectomy or radiation therapy alone. In terms of the surgical options, there are different forms of prostatectomies. These options include open, laparoscopic, and minimally invasive or robotic-assisted surgeries. Graefen and colleagues[26] elucidated on the fact that research suggests that there are few to no differences in terms of the oncologic outcomes among the surgical practices. Many of the reported differences may stem from prior experience and expertise performing such operations.[26] Some patients opt for minimally invasive interventions compared with radiation or surgery. Ultrasound therapy is one such intervention that has shown interesting clinical progress. The treatment is not as effective as conventional invasive techniques, and Bass and colleagues[27] demonstrated that high-intensity focused ultrasound therapy was not able to assist all intermediate or high-risk groups given that 49% of patients had local recurrence. Although high-intensity focused ultrasound therapy had a high failure rate, it is very clear that the negative side effects were minimal and inconsequential.[27]

Another therapy to discuss is the androgen deprivation therapy. Hormonal manipulation is effective in treating local prostate cancer because the tumor is still castrate sensitive. LHRH agonist affects the hormonal balances in the production of gonadotropin releasing hormone and its effect on the production of testosterone in the testes. There are several LHRH agonists, including leuprorelin, goserelin, and triptorelin. Comparison for the effectiveness of LHRH agonists, goserelin, triptorelin, and leuprolide in treating prostate cancer showed significant differences in the castration levels at less than 10 ng/dL, whereas the efficacy was comparable at 20 ng/dL or higher doses.[28]

When prostate cancer is in its advanced stages and has become resistant to hormonal therapy, this is known as the castrate-resistant phase. Patients usually present with CRPC. Abiraterone and enzalutamide are 2 vital drugs that are used to treat patients presenting with this form of prostate cancer. A study conducted by Hahn and colleagues[29] found that androgen deprivation therapy in combination with abiraterone showed significant improvement in overall survival and promising cancer-free survival after 3 years. Furthermore, Cornford and colleagues[30] highlighted the benefits of enzalutamide on numerous clinical determinants for improved course of prostate cancer.

As second-generation drugs lose effectiveness and potency in the fight against prostate cancer, adjuvant chemotherapies seem to be the last resort. Docetaxel is a common taxane used for metastasis. Although it is used in combination with the aforementioned treatments for improved efficacy of therapeutic intensity and delivery, docetaxel has not been shown to be effective after radical prostatectomy.[31] Cursano and colleagues[32] look at how combinations of radium-223 with docetaxel and cabazitaxel affected patients who had bone metastases. Strikingly different clinical outcomes have emerged from this study, which warrants the need to investigate the effects of these combinations.

Novel agents that are used to treat prostate cancer include the use of proxalutamide, an androgen receptor antagonist. Furthermore, nanoparticles are being developed to enhance delivery of chemotherapeutic agents such as docetaxel. The potency of docetaxel and doxorubicin was increased by enhancing their codelivery using nanocarriers.[33] Furthermore, Hammer and colleagues[34] describe how a novel antibody-based therapy called thorium-227 may be helpful in targeting prostate-specific membrane antigen (PSMA) and alleviating metastatic CRPC.

IMMUNOTHERAPY IN CANCER

Over the past decades, the conventional strategies for cancer treatment include surgery, chemotherapy, and radiotherapy. The concept that the immune system can recognize and control tumor growth was first report in 1891 by William Coley, who demonstrated that bacterial toxins cause antitumor immune responses in some patients, particularly sarcomas,[35] but with limited clinical efficacy. After that, immunotherapy has become an appealing strategy for various types of tumors. Different cancer immunotherapy approaches have proven efficacy,[36] such as cell-based therapies, monoclonal antibodies, cancer vaccinations, and even immune checkpoint blockade therapy.

Later in the 1960s, Thomas and Burnet[37] put forward the theory of cancer immune surveillance. According to this theory, the body's immune system would use tumor-associated antigens to eliminate malignant cells.[37] It took about one-half of a century for this theory to be accepted.[38] In the 1990s, it was demonstrated that the CD8-positive T lymphocytes had the ability to kill tumor cells that presented antigens for melanocyte differentiation.[39] It was also demonstrated that the absence of interferon gamma led to incidence of sarcoma and lung cancer in mice.[40] A subsequent study was done to assess the role of T cells in antitumor immune responses, that ultimately led to the use of IL-2, a T-cell growth factor, in clinics. Briefly, tumor-infiltrating lymphocytes (TILs) from patients were activated with IL-2 in vitro, which was subsequently injected to patient.[41] The US Food and Drug Administration (FDA) later approved IL-2 in 1991 for treating metastatic renal cell carcinoma. However, IL-2 treatments had some caveats. The response rate was relatively low with high toxicity, underlining the need to improve immunotherapeutic strategies.[42,43]

In 1975, monoclonal antibodies were made with the development of the hybridoma technology.[44] Subsequently, treatments using monoclonal antibody started evolving and rituximab was the first FDA-approved drug for treating B-cell lymphomas. This drug is a monoclonal antibody that targets the CD20 antigen, expressed ubiquitously in B cells. This treatment brings about cell death as a result of cytotoxicity, the activation of complements and induction of apoptosis.[45,46] During the same era, chimeric antigen receptor (CAR) T cells were also developed, which had the ability to combine the self-renewal and cytolytic capacity of T cells with the antigen-binding properties of antibodies.[47,48] CAR T cells are chimeric fusion proteins that express an extracellular domain that has the antigen recognition ability, including single chain variable fragments, which are derived from the antibody, and the T-cell activation end domains. In CAR T-cell therapy, the CD8$^+$ T cells of a patient are manipulated ex vivo to elicit an immune response when subsequently reinfused into the patient. The most promising results was seen with CAR T cells targeting CD19 in hematologic malignancies.[49,50] Two FDA-approved CART19 therapies are tisagenlecleucel and axicabtagene ciloleucel.[51–54]

Checkpoints have channelized immune response to pathogens as well as self-antigens. Memory T cells as well as cytokine secretion in addition to an individual's CD8$^+$ cytotoxic T lymphocyte (CTL) cells are required to activate immune response at cellular level. Ligands like CD80 or CD86 bind to CD28 and the CD28 gets replaced by CTL antigen 4 (CTLA)-4, which send inhibitory signals on the T-cell surface. This leads to switching off of the signal or a checkpoint being applied.

Cancer cells express increased levels of CTLA-4. The other inhibitory mechanism in cancer cells is between antigen-presenting cells (APCs) and programmed death 1 (PD-1) and PD ligand 1 (PD-L1)/PD-L2 leading to inactivation by programmed death of CTLs. Over recent years, several antibodies that target cellular immune checkpoints (eg, PD-1/PD-L1 and CTLA-4) were developed to promote the activation of T-cell and tumor regression. This therapeutic strategy has demonstrated benefits in tumors having a high mutation burden, enabling tumor-mutated antigens (neoantigens) to enter stage in cancer immunotherapy.[55–61] In patients with melanoma, blockage of both PD-1 and CTLA4 lead to better survival.

However, CAR T cells and checkpoint blockade are not always effective, mainly owing to the immune suppressive environment locally created by the cancer. Further several cytokines with immunosuppressive properties are occasionally turned on by the cancer cells. This facilitates the cancer cells to attract regulatory T cells and myeloid-derived suppressor cells that have the ability to block autoimmunity. Regulatory T cells act by suppressing B-cell Ig production and activation.[62–65] So therapeutic antibodies targeting regulatory T cells and myeloid-derived suppressor cells in combination with checkpoint inhibitors or CAR T cells show promise.

IMMUNOTHERAPY IN GENITOURINARY CANCERS

Genitourinary malignancies represent a heterogeneous group of diseases, such as kidney cancer, bladder cancer, and prostate cancer. Treatment of those diseases involves surgery, radiation, and systemic therapy. Immunotherapies have been used in genitourinary cancers with promising clinical benefits and outcomes.

Kidney cancer lead to more than 175,000 deaths in 2018, and there is a constant increase in its incidence worldwide.[66] In the United States, it is the eighth most common cancer, with an estimated number of 73,750 for new cancer cases and estimated deaths of 14,830 in 2020.[1] Among the different subtypes of kidney cancer, the most prevalent form is the clear cell renal cell carcinoma and represents about 60% to 80% of all the primary kidney cancers.[67]

Studies showed the association between the immune system and kidney cancer.[68,69] For kidney cancer, cytokines have been used as immunotherapies for more than a decade. In 10% to 25% of patients with kidney cancer, the cytokines interferon-alpha and IL-2 improved objective response rates and provided sustained remissions in a subset of the patients.[70–72] For a long time, IL-12 was the first-line therapy for advanced kidney cancer, but because it has severe side effects, it is no longer a treatment of choice. In addition to cytokines and targeted therapies, several new types of immunotherapy have become important in the treatment of kidney cancer. The most notable immune checkpoint inhibitors are those that block the functions of CTLA-4 and PD-1. CTLA-4 helps to decrease the inflammatory T-cell response by facilitating the activated T cells to be disengaged.[73] The CTLA-4–blocking antibody ipilimumab showed partial response.[74] Treatment with nivolumab, the anti PD-1 antibody, showed treatment response in 27% patients with RCC, making nivolumab a treatment of choice.[75] However, current studies indicate that single agent immunotherapy may not benefit all patients, highlighting the need for combined treatment strategies to improve efficacy.

Atezolizumab is a monoclonal antibody against PD-L1. Bevacizumab is a vascular endothelial growth factor inhibitor. The combination treatment with Atezolizumab and bevacizumab potentiates PD-L1 inhibition.[76,77] In a phase II trial on treatment-naïve patients with metastatic RCC, better antitumor activity was demonstrated with combination therapy with atezolizumab plus bevacizumab compared with atezolizumab alone or sunitinib alone. In PD-L1 patients treated with combination therapy, a higher progression-free survival was reported.[78] Another trial (IMmotion 151) demonstrated that combination therapy had a longer progression-free survival and improved objective response rates in PD-L1–expressing patients.[79] Avelumab (anti–PD-L1) combined with axitinib (vascular endothelial growth factor inhibitor) showed superior progression-free survival (13.8 months vs 7.2 months).[80]

A clinical trial in phase Ib for the use of pembrolizumab (an anti–PD-1 agent) with axitinib (an anti-vascular endothelial growth factor agent) demonstrated promising antitumor activity; 73% patients achieved an objective as well as similar toxicity of each monotherapy.[81] A phase III study comparing axitinib plus pembrolizumab with sunitinib monotherapy (NCT02853331) is ongoing to further evaluate whether or not the combination works better than a vascular endothelial growth factor inhibitor monotherapy. Compared with the group treated with sunitinib, the combination group demonstrated significantly longer overall survival, longer progression-free survival, an improved objective response rate, and a prolonged response.[82]

IMMUNOTHERAPY IN BLADDER CANCER

In the United States, bladder cancer is the fifth most common cancer, with estimated new cancer cases of 81,400 and estimated deaths of 17,980 in 2020.[1] Immunotherapy for bladder cancer has a long history. Both early and advanced stages of bladder cancer has been treated with different immunotherapies, including bacillus of Calmette and Guerin (BCG) intravesical immunotherapy[83,84] and anti–PD-1/PD-L1 immune checkpoint blockade.

BCG has been applied to treat patients with non–muscle invasive bladder cancer since 1976.[85] In addition, BCG was the first immunotherapy developed for non–muscle invasive bladder cancer approved by the FDA. BCG suppresses the tumor cell growth by infiltrating the bladder with inflammatory cells and upregulating cytokines. BCG immunotherapy was superior to various intravesical chemotherapy drugs and was more effective in preventing tumor recurrence.[86–91] However, BCG treatment failed in approximately 40% of patients with non–muscle invasive bladder cancer.[92] This is a main problem that requires alternative strategies.

There are other FDA-approved immunotherapy options for bladder cancer, including PD-1/PD-L1 inhibitors, including atezolizumab,[93] durvalumab,[94] avelumab,[95] nivolumab,[96] and pembrolizumab.[97]

Anti–programmed Death Ligand 1 Immunotherapies

The first anti–PD-L1 antibody to be tested in bladder cancer immunotherapy was atezolizumab, which was approved by the FDA in 2014.[98] Atezolizumab showed good activity in metastatic urothelial bladder cancer, which was associated with positive PD-L1, had significantly higher response rates. A multicenter phase II trial of atezolizumab showed an improved overall objective response rate compared with a historical platinum-based chemotherapy control (15% vs 10%).[93] A postprogression study from Imvigor210 also demonstrated that platinum-treated patients with either locally advanced or with metastatic urothelial carcinoma still benefited from continued atezolizumab treatment.[99]

After the success of atezolizumab, durvalumab, another anti–PD-L1 drug, was tested in advanced bladder cancer.[94] Durvalumab, an engineered human antibody that selectively blocks the binding of PDL-1 to PD-1 and CD80, demonstrated encouraging clinical activity in locally advanced/metastatic bladder patients with cancer.[94]

Avelumab is the third anti–PD-L1 inhibitor approved for locally advanced or metastatic bladder cancer with disease progression. Avelumab is a fully humanized antibody developed against PDL-1 that assists in using the immune response of the human body against the cancer. Avelumab successfully showed a significant improvement in overall survival.

Anti–programmed Death 1 Immunotherapies

Nivolumab, a PD-1–blocking antibody, demonstrated safety and efficacy in locally advanced or metastatic urothelial carcinoma.[96,100] Nivolumab demonstrated antitumor activity and survival in the global population.[101]

Another highly selective humanized monoclonal antibody, pembrolizumab, blocks the interaction between PD-1 and PD-L1/PDL-2. Compared with chemotherapy, pembrolizumab demonstrated better response in all patient and also in patients having PD-L1–positive score of 10% or higher. Compared with the chemotherapy group, the median overall survival of the pembrolizumab-treated group was significantly longer.[102] Pembrolizumab has been approved by FDA as a second-line therapy after platinum treatment and as a first-line therapy for patients with locally advanced/metastatic urothelial carcinoma that are ineligible for cisplatin treatment.

Testicular Germ Cell Tumors

The majority of patients with metastatic germ cell tumors could be cured with first-line or salvage chemotherapy.[103] However, a group of 15% to 20% patients who failed after those treatment need develop additional therapeutic options.[104] Recent targeted therapies trials did not show promising efficiency.

IMMUNOTHERAPY FOR METASTATIC PROSTATE CANCER

Immunotherapy is a growing area of research for prostate cancer, given the importance and need for alternative treatments. Immunotherapy fundamentally encompass harnessing and exploitation of the patient's individual immune system to fight against the cancer. Augmenting the strength of the immune system by inducing specific interactions to take place between T cells and their compliment antigens on cancer cells may prove to be useful in the targeted destruction of tumors. Furthermore, immune checkpoint pathway CTLA-4/B7 inhibitors like ipilimumab, tremelimumab, and prostvac, as well as PD-1 pathway inhibitors such as nivolumab, pembrolizumab, and pidilizumab are specific types of drugs that may be helpful in boosting an immune response that was initially suppressed by the growth and spread of cancer.

Although several immunotherapies have been FDA approved for metastatic castration-resistant prostate cancer, there is still a major lack of efficient use of immunotherapeutic agents for this disease. This is mainly because prostate cancer for a prolonged period of time has been conceived to be an immune desert. Unlike other solid tumors, prostate has never shown a strong immune infiltrate within the tumor. Further, prostate tumors present a tumor microenvironment that is metabolically hostile, with increased glycolysis. This environment suppresses T-cell function. Further, tumor-infiltrating T cells also have a reduced mitochondrial function.[105] Tumor immune score is computed based on the TIL expression within the tumor. This along with the tumor specific inflammatory gene signature is used to categorize tumors as "hot" or "cold."[106] Unlike other solid tumors like urothelial and lung cancers, prostate tumors have more immunosuppressive factors than immunostimulatory factors leading to an impaired TIL activity. However, studies that looked for other T-cell populations report increased expression of CD4$^+$ and CD8$^+$ forkhead box P3 (Foxp3$^+$) regulatory T cells in tumors.[107,108] Further, a study also reports that increased Foxp3+ TILs were associated with worse survival outcomes.[109] Besides immunosuppressive lymphocytes, protolerogenic tumor-associated macrophage has been reported to be infiltrated in high numbers in prostate cancer tumor microenvironment.[110] M2-associated cytokines and chemokines that are immunosuppressive are also secreted along with transforming growth factor-β2, by the macrophages. So, some studies have elucidated the need for targeting transforming growth factor-β before checkpoint inhibition to get better therapeutic benefit.[111]

Prostate cancer has a low tumor mutation burden, which results in low neoantigen expression compared with other tumor types.[112] As a result, immunotherapy is speculated to be less effective. Despite having a low somatic alteration burden, prostate cancer does present with a high number of DNA damage and repair gene defects.[8,113,114] Mutations in DNA damage and repair genes especially in members of the homologous recombination repair pathway both somatic and germline, makes prostate cancer immune sensitive. So prostate cancer cannot be called a cold tumor or an immune desert.

The various immunotherapies that have been tested on prostate cancer can be broadly classified into vaccines, cell therapies, checkpoint blockade therapies, oncolytic virus therapy, and targeted antibodies.

Cancer Vaccines

Vaccines are composed of an adjuvant that can activate APCs like dendritic cells, as well as a target protein that is associated with the cancer.[115] Using the patient's own dendritic cells that are pulsed with tumor antigens, is an approach that has lot of popularity in the vaccine world. Peptides from tumor antigens are used to pulse dendritic cells and have shown good response in preclinical models.[116] Therapeutic cancer vaccines that facilitate the body's immune system to recognize tumor-associated antigens and generate a T-cell response have shown considerable success in prostate cancer. Prostate cancer is a promising target for vaccine-based therapy owing to the expression of several specific tumor-associated antigens like PSA and PSMA, as well as prostatic acid phosphatase.[117]

Sipuleucel-T

Interest in immunotherapy has gained momentum with the relative success of the FDA-approved treatment of sipuleucel-T. Sipuleucel-T, an autologous vaccine, has been derived from peripheral dendritic cell collection by leukapheresis. This collection of cells is stimulated by PA2024, a fusion protein of an immune-activating cytokine, granulocyte-macrophage colony-stimulated factor linked to the target antigen, prostatic acid phosphatase.[118,119] After 36 to 44 hours, the dendritic cells, which are now primed, are reinfused back into the patient for generating a CD4$^+$ and CD8$^+$ T-cell response that is prostatic acid phosphatase specific.[120,121] This process is repeated 3 times at 2-week intervals over the course of 1 month to complete the full course of therapy.[122]

Sipuleucel-T was the first immunotherapy to be approved by FDA for patients with metastatic CRPC. The IMPACT trial randomized patients in 2:1 fashion and received 3 doses of sipuleucel-T or of placebo. This study demonstrated a improvement in median overall survival by 4.1 months and a 22% decrease in the risk of death.[118] Despite the beneficial effect of sipuleucel-T, several other prostate cancer vaccines that were tested in phase III trials have not been that promising.

GVAX

Another cell-based vaccine, GVAX, has been synthesized using prostate cancer cell lines, LNCaP and PC3, by transducing with a retrovirus that was made replication defective and had also been modified genetically to be able to bear granulocyte-macrophage colony-stimulated factor and bring about the recruitment of APC to the injection site.[123,124] Although an initial phase I/II trial in hormone-naïve patients with prostate

cancer with relapse in PSA, showed promising results,[125] 2 subsequent phase III clinical trials (VITAL-1 and VITAL-2) did not show significant benefit and so were terminated early. In the VITAL-1 trial, randomization of patients with asymptomatic metastatic CRPC was done to receive either GVAX or docetaxel-prednisone. Initial analysis showed that less than 30% of patients would meet the primary end point, which was overall survival, and so the trial was terminated early. In contrast, the phase III trial, VITAL-2, on symptomatic taxane naïve metastatic CRPC patients who received GVAX alone or GVAX plus docetaxel/prednisone, also terminated early as a result of increased mortality among patients in the intervention group.

The flaws in the trial design could have possibly led to the negative outcomes. There was no placebo control in the study. Moreover, before the phase II trial VITAL-2, the recommended doses for the combination therapy of GVAX and docetaxel were not determined, which may have also contributed to experimental flaws.[121,126]

PROSTVAC

PROSTVAC is also another vaccine that includes in viral vectors PSA gene and several T-cell costimulatory molecules. It creates a heterologous prime boost by combining recombinant fowlpox and vaccinia virus.[127] This vaccine infects APCs to generate cell surface proteins expressed on the surface of APCs finally leading to tumor cell destruction as a result of interaction of APCs with the T cells.[127] PROSTVAC has been used in several clinical trials. An increase in PSA progression-free survival was seen in 63% of the patients for a period of 6 months. Furthermore, the phase II trial showed a significant reduction of the PSA doubling.[128] Other studies have been established using PROSTVAC. In another phase II study, patients with minimally symptomatic metastatic CRPC were included in the study and were randomized to either receive the vaccine or placebo. Even though the study showed negative results for its primary end point (progression-free survival), overall survival was seen to be significantly increased.[129] PROSTVAC has shown no effect on overall survival in patients with metastatic CRPC.[130]

Polyinosinic-polycytidylic acid and poly-L-lysine

Although the capacity to activate a T-cell response has been tested for several dendritic cell-based vaccines, their effects has been limited. Polyinosinic-polycytidylic acid, and poly-L-lysine, an immunostimulant, is a double-stranded RNA complex that acts like a viral mimic. It is composed of poly-L-lysine double-stranded RNA and carboxymethylcellulose, polyinosinic-polycytidylic acid. It activates dendritic cells by binding to toll-like receptor 3, MDA5, and other pathogen receptors.[131–133] The synergy between MDA5 and toll-like receptor 3 activation makes Poly IC a superior vaccine. Toll-like receptor 3 contributes to CD8[+] T-cell activation and MDA5 is required for the survival of CD8 memory T cells. Poly-ICLC (Hiltonol®) is being tested in several clinical trials as an immune stimulant.

There are 4 clinical trials for Poly ICLC in prostate cancer. Out of the 2 completed studies, 1 trial tested PSMA and TARP peptide vaccine in combination with Poly IC-LC in HLA-A2[+] patients with rising PSA (NCT00694551), and the other tested combination therapies of Poly IC LC with MUC1 vaccine in patients with advanced prostate cancer (NCT00374049). One of the studies at our institute is testing IT/IM Poly-IC LC in patients with high-risk, clinically localized prostate cancer (NCT03262103).

Checkpoint Inhibition Therapy

Another type of drug is the immune checkpoint inhibitor that blocks proteins on the immune cells. This drug assists in making the immune system more effective at destroying cancer cells. They function by releasing inhibitory responses that regulate T-cell–mediated immunity. Immune checkpoints are inhibitory mechanism of immune cells used to regulate immune response. Antibodies blocking immune checkpoint receptors and that are approved for clinical use include the CTLA-4 as well as PD-1 and its ligand PD-L1.

The first successful immune checkpoint inhibitor to receive FDA approval was anti–CTLA-4 (ipilimumab).[134] Ipilimumab was also the first immune checkpoint that was studied in prostate cancer. CTLA4 controls T-cell activation and competes with CD28, the costimulatory receptor, for ligand binding, to CD80 and CD86. This leads to translocation and expression of CTLA4 on the cell surface of T cells. CTLA-4 pathway blockade was achieved using a fully human monoclonal antibody called ipilimumab.[135] Another phase III clinical trial in metastatic CRPC patients who had progressed on docetaxel-chemotherapy was randomized to receive either ipilimumab or placebo after bone-directed radiotherapy. Although there was no benefit in the primary end point of overall survival, some benefit was observed in progression-free survival with ipilimumab over placebo. There was a significant reduction in the PSA in patients who were treated with ipilimumab. Additionally, a greater benefit was also seen in subset of patients,

such as lower alkaline phosphatase concentrations, higher hemoglobin concentrations, and finally absence of visceral metastases. The median overall survival was significantly higher with ipilimumab compared with placebo.[136,137]

Pembrolizumab (Keytruda) has been shown effective for a low rate hypermutated subtype of prostate cancers.[138] The effects of pembrolizumab were studied on a large group of patients who had metastatic CRPC. They were divided into cohorts 1, 2, and 3 based on if they were PD-L1 positive, PD-L1 negative, or bone predominant, respectively. Treatment with 200 mg of pembrolizumab showed that median overall survival was highest for cohort 3 at 14.1 months and the estimated 12-month survival rates were 41% for cohort 1%, 35% for cohort 2%, and 62% for cohort 3. This study warrants the need to further research the effects of pembrolizumab on bone-predominant disease.[139,140]

PD-1 is also expressed on activated immune cells including B cells, T cells, and natural killer cells. PD-1 has a tyrosine-based inhibitory motif and also an immune-receptor tyrosine-based switch motif that gets phosphorylated when it binds to the B7 ligands PD-L1 or PD-L2. This caused SH2 domain containing tyrosine phosphatase 2 to be recruited and finally leads to inhibition of T-cell proliferation. PD-L1 is expressed on APCs, T cells, vascular endothelial cells, stromal cells, and cancer cells.[141,142] PD-L1 expression is induced owing to production of inflammatory cytokines, interleukins (IL-2, IL-7, and IL-15), when antigens expressed by MHC complex get presented to T cells. T-cell effector functions are inhibited owing to PD-1/PD-L1 interactions through distinct mechanisms compared with CTLA-4.[143,144] Antibody-based blockade of the PD-1 receptor or its ligand increases the antitumor immunity and tumor growth suppression.[144] The PD-1/PD-L1 pathway is activated in several tumor types such as in the lung, kidney, and bladder.[145] It is clear that early phase clinical trials that are investigating nivolumab (PD-1 blockade) and prostate cancer have shown very small success and that further research experiments are needed to investigate these complex biochemical mechanisms Studies of nivolumab monotherapy, showed no measurable responses.[75,134,146,147] These studies demonstrate that the success of immune checkpoint inhibitors in patients with metastatic CRPC has been limited,[59,75,134] expect for some isolated response seen in patients having mutations in either BRCA 1/2, CDK12, or microsatellite instability–high mutations. Ipilimumab has been FDA approved as a drug therapy for metastatic melanoma and has shown potential in treatment for other types of cancers like renal, lung, and prostate. Currently, combination therapies using ipilimumab would be more useful in the treatment of metastatic CRPC as opposed to treatment alone. Nevertheless, studies have illustrated that the response rates to ipilimumab have ranged in the 10% to 15% range, further supporting the notion that it is not a completely effective therapy.

More in-depth and comprehensive research is needed to assist the immune system recognize prostate tumors and as well as activating the immune cells for targeted destruction of the cancer. Various studies are looking at whether combinations of immunotherapy drugs may be more effective in treating prostate cancer compared with single immunotherapies.

Adoptive Cell Therapy

In this form of treatment, the immune cells of the body are geared toward eliminating cancer. The immune cells are either isolated and expanded or genetically engineered to improve their ability to fight cancer. Cell therapy include TIL therapy, T cell therapy, CAR T-cell therapy, as well as natural killer cell therapy.

In TIL therapy, the T cells from the tumors are expanded in the presence of IL-2 and reinfused into the patients.[148] TIL therapy has been successful in melanoma as well as other solid tumors. Recent studies have also demonstrated the ability of using TIL therapy for patients with prostate cancer.[149]

In both T-cell therapy and CAR T-cell therapy, the T cells from patients are genetically modified ex vivo, expanded, and readministered to the patient. In T-cell therapy, the T cells from the patient are genetically modified to be able to target specific cancer antigens, whereas in CAR T-cell therapies, the patients T cells are coupled with synthetic receptors, CAR. CAR T-cell therapy is advantageous over the other adoptive cell therapies mainly because CARs can bind to the cancer cells even if their antigens are not presented on cell surface. However, 1 disadvantage with CAR T-cell therapy is that the range of potential antigen targets are limited, owing to the intercellular expression of most proteins, which makes them unavailable for CARs.

For effective CAR T-cell therapy in prostate cancer, the most critical step is the identification of tumor-associated antigens that are constitutively expressed by the cancer cells. The proteins that have been used as TAAs for prostate cancer CAR T cell therapy are mainly PSA, prostatic acid phosphatase, prostate stem cell antigen (PSCA), PSMA, and epithelial cell adhesion molecule. Of these, PSMA and PSCA are the CAR T-cell targeted antigens that have been mostly used in metastatic prostate cancer. In the phase III trials of sipuleucel-T for metastatic CRPC patients, the antigen presenting cells were pre-exposed to human granulocyte macrophage colony stimulating factor and prostatic acid phosphatase fused protein.[149] PSCA is another cell surface glycoprotein expressed in prostate cells. CTL response HLA-A2 restricted anti-PSCA peptides has been evaluated in vitro in several studies.[150–152] CTL response has also been studied in TRAMP mouse models vaccinated with PSCA-encoded viral vectors.[153,154] Further in xenograft models prostate cancer inhibition has been evaluated using anti-PSCA antibodies.[155–157] PSMA, a transmembrane glycoprotein, shows higher expression in high grade prostate tumors. Invitro studied have demonstrated CTL response using HLA-2–restricted PSMA peptides.[158–161] In several recent studies, chimeric anti-PSMA immunoglobulin T-cell receptor constructs have been used to promote a T-cell response. In mouse models PSMA-CAR T cells were able to abolish metastatic prostate cancer.[162] PSMA CAR T-cells coupled with CD28 showed significant decrease in tumor volume in mice.[163] In another study anti-PSMA CAR T cells resistant to transforming growth factor-β caused cell lysis of PSMA expressing cells with an increase of interferon-γ, IL-2, and CD8$^+$ cells.[164]

CAR T-cell therapy shows promise mainly in preclinical studies on metastatic prostate cancer. However, more investigation on risk to patients is essential to develop plans for management of toxicity. Further among all the TAAs the one that's most safe an effective is yet to be determined.

Oncolytic Virus Therapy

Immunotherapies are currently used to activate the immune system enabling it to target and kill the cancer cells. These new drugs can enhance and facilitate antitumor activity by promoting the function of specific cells, such as the T cells and natural killer cells. However, recent studies have suggested that, even with the use of these immunotherapies, cancer cells can adapt to the environment, evade the immune system, and induce immunosuppression. Therefore, oncolytic viruses have been proposed as a novel method to counteract this tumor-associated immunosuppression and evasion. Oncolytic viruses have even been shown to potentiate the effectiveness of several immunotherapeutic approaches that involve immune checkpoint inhibition. Therefore, it is important to consider the potential applications and practical usefulness of oncolytic viruses in combination with other drugs and immunotherapies in targeting metastatic prostate cancer.[165]

Viruses typically work by infecting cells through the injection and incorporation of their DNA or RNA elements into the host's genetic machinery. Therefore, viruses can be used to target specific cancer cells that may be susceptible and vulnerable to such molecular modification. Cancer cells may not have protective qualities that allow for antiviral defense mechanisms. As such, the development of specific oncolytic viruses that target cancer cells, as opposed to healthy cells, can potentially induce antitumor responses. Furthermore, oncolytic viruses can potentially induce a lytic reaction in the cancer cells in which the multiplication and growth of progeny in the host cells eventually induces a burst effect. In conjunction with immunotherapeutic stimulation of the immune cells, this effect may help in synergistically eliminating tumor growth.[166]

Viral infection occurs because the virus recognizes its target cell based on cellular surface receptors. One oncolytic virus that was engineered from the herpes simplex virus is called T-VEC. T-VEC is able to recognize surface receptors such as the herpesvirus entry mediator, nectin-1, and nectin-2.[167] Engineering these oncolytic viruses can allow researchers to manipulate them in very specific ways. For example, current research involves the modification of their receptors for entry into cancer cells as well as restriction and deletion of certain viral protein expression via oncogenic promoter function.[168] In the context of prostate cancer, oncolytic viruses have been engineered to involve a PSA or a PSA promoter. Effectively, this leads to E1A expression and viral proliferation specific to prostate cancer cells.[169]

One study investigated the role of using virotherapy in inhibiting prostate cancer growth and metastasis. An oncolytic adenovirus, ZD55, was developed to target SATB1. ZD55-SATB1 inhibited both viability and invasion in prostate cancer cell lines.[170] Another study aimed to understand how oncolytic rhabdovirus VSV-GP functioned as a therapeutic modality in prostate cancer cells. VSV-GP infected 6 out of 7 prostate cancer cell lines and the mouse models achieved long-term remission. Several of the cancer cell lines developed resistance to interferon type I, suggesting a reduced antiviral responses.[171]

Targeted Antibodies

Another immunotherapy that has been shown to be effective in eliminating cancer cells involves targeted antibodies. Antibodies are proteins naturally produced from mature B cells. Antibodies can precisely target, bind to cell surfaces, and disrupt pathogenic cancer cell activity. After the antibodies bind to the cell surface of the cancer cells, immune cells can recognize them and induce different immune mechanisms.[172] Several different classifications of targeted antibodies include monoclonal antibodies, bispecific antibodies, and antibody–drug conjugation.

One study evaluated the efficacy of a specifically engineered antibody–drug conjugate called MEDI3726. This molecule contains an antibody called J591 that specifically binds to PSMA presented on cancer cell surfaces. Cancer cells typically have increased surface expression of PSMA making this a very attractive biotarget for tumor-mediated destruction. Also, MED13726 has another element called the pyrrolobenzodiazepine dimer tesirine that is, conjugated to the anti-PSMA antibody. As the antibody binds to PSMA express on cancer surface membranes, the entire MEDI3726 is engulfed into a vesicle and incorporated into the tumor cell. Pyrrolobenzodiazepine subsequently dissociated from the drug and binds to DNA and leads to cell death. MEDI3726 has shown potential as it led to specific cytotoxicity and antitumor activity in prostate cancer cell lines.[173]

Several studies have illustrated the efficacy of using monoclonal antibodies to target cancer cells. For example, it was found that N-cadherin expression is increased in metastatic tumors of individuals with CRPC. Administering monoclonal antibodies that targeted the ectodomain of N-cadherin effectively reduced proliferation and growth of prostate cancer cells in CRPC xenografts.[174] Another molecule upregulated in prostate cancer is TRIM24. A study revealed that silencing TRIM24 through a human monoclonal PSMA antibody-mediated TRIM24 small interfering RNA, drastically suppressed proliferation and invasion of the PSMA-positive CRPC cells.[175]

Furthermore, bispecific antibodies are used to recognize both the receptor on the surface of T cells as well as the specific tumor antigens. Thus, this antibody bridges the 2 cells together, which activates the T cells. TSAxCD28 bispecifics for targeting prostate cancer malignancy shows promising tolerance in immunocompetent mouse models and minor toxicity.[176] Also, 3E10-AR441 bispecific antibodies were developed and blocked genomic signaling of androgen receptor in LNCaP cells and inhibited prostate cancer cell growth under androgen-simulated conditions.[177] In xenograft models, AMG 160, a bispecific antibody that targets PSMA expressing prostate cancer cells and CD3 of T cells, caused significant decrease in tumor growth.[178] **Fig. 1** gives a representation of current and emerging therapies for metastatic prostate cancer. Further, in **Table 1**, we summarize some of the recent clinical trials for immunotherapies in metastatic prostate cancer.

PRECLINICAL MODELS FOR IMMUNOTHERAPY RESEARCH FOR METASTATIC PROSTATE CANCER

With a revolution in development of therapies that harness the immune response of tumors, the need to develop preclinical models that replicate the disease and can be used to test novel immunotherapies becomes extremely important. However, developing a preclinical model that can appropriately recapitulate the disease and help test the efficacy of immunotherapy is extremely challenging.

Cell Line Models

Several cell lines have been used to study to model immunotherapy for prostate cancer. The RM1, RM-9 murine prostate cancer cells were derived from ras and myc transformed mouse prostate reconstitution C57BL/6 mice model.[179,180] Syngeneic prostate cancer model from gp100-transfected murine RM1 cells has complete immunity and can be used to evaluate CD8+ lymphocyte-mediated antitumor immunity.[181] The combination of nitroxoline and PD-1 blockade in RM9-Luc-PSA mouse model can significantly enhance antitumor immunity by increasing CD44+CD62L+CD8+ memory T cells and reducing myeloid-derived suppressor cells.[182]

Transgenic adenocarcinoma mouse prostate (TRAMP)-C1, TRAMP-C2, and TRAMP-C3 were derived from a TRAMP model. Both TRAMP-C1 and TRAMP-C2 are tumorigenic, whereas TRAMP-C3 easily grows in vitro but does not form tumors.[183] Dexamethasone plus octreotide enhances the antitumor efficiency of docetaxel in a TRAMP-C1 prostate cancer model.[184] TRAMP-C1 cells showed increased expression of CXCL16 after radiation therapy, indicating a radiotherapy combination with immunotherapy.[185]

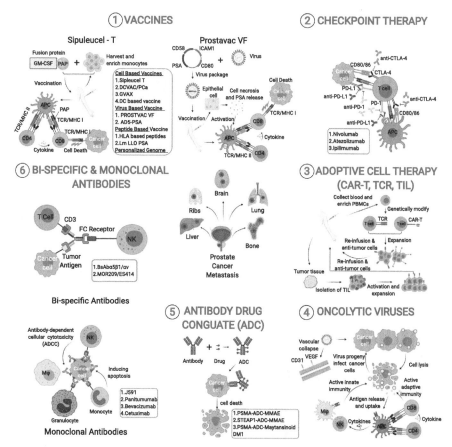

Fig. 1. Current and emerging therapies for metastatic prostate cancer. Clockwise from top left, vaccines, checkpoint therapy, adoptive cell therapy, oncolytic viruses, antibody–drug conjugate and bispecific and monoclonal antibodies.

Table 1
Current clinical trials testing novel immunotherapies for metastatic prostate cancer

Trial Number	Drug	Phase	Tumor Type	Mechanism of Action
NCT03834506[179]	Pembrolizumab + docetaxel	Phase III	Metastatic CRPC	Pembrolizumab targets the cellular pathway of proteins found on immune cells and cancer cells, known as PD-1/PD-L1.
NCT03834519[180]	Pembrolizumab + olaparib vs abiraterone acetate or enzalutamide	Phase III	Metastatic CRPC	Pembrolizumab targets the cellular pathway of proteins found on immune cells and cancer cells, known as PD-1/PD-L1.
NCT04262154[181]	Abiraterone, atezolizumab, lupron, and radiation therapy	Phase II	Metastatic hormone-sensitive prostate cancer	Atezolizumab is a monoclonal antibody of IgG1 isotype against the protein PD-L1.
NCT04104893[182]	Pembrolizumab	Phase II	Metastatic castrate resistant prostate cancer	Pembrolizumab targets the cellular pathway of proteins found on immune cells and cancer cells, known as PD-1/PD-L1.
NCT03693612[183]	GSK3359609 and tremelimumab	Phase II	Castrate-resistant prostate adenocarcinoma	GSK3359609 is an anti-Inducible T cell co-stimulator receptor agonist antibody. Tremelimumab is a fully human monoclonal antibody against CTLA-4.
NCT03575819[184]	FOR46	Phase I	Metastatic CRPC	FOR 46, an antibody–drug conjugate targeting CD46 protein.
NCT03577028[185]	HPN424	Phase I	Metastatic CRPC	HPN424 targets PSMA.
NCT02985957[186]	Nivolumab + ipilimumab or cabazitaxel	Phase II	Metastatic CRPC	Nivolumab blocks cancer cells' protective proteins against T cells.
NCT03972657[187]	REGN5678 + cemiplimab	Phase I/II	Metastatic CRPC	Cemiplimab targets PD-1 so it acts as a checkpoint inhibitor.
NCT04227275[188]	CART-PSMA-TGFβRDN	Phase I	Metastatic CRPC	Co-expression of TGFβRdn on PSMA-redirected CAR T cells increase T-cell proliferation and greater tumor eradication.
NCT03725761[189]	Sacituzumab govitecan	Phase II	Metastatic CRPC	Sacituzumab govitecan targets the Trop-2 receptor that helps the cancer to grow, divide, and spread.
NCT03554317[190]	Testosterone cypionate and nivolumab	Phase II	Metastatic CRPC	Nivolumab blocks cancer cells' protective proteins against T cells.
NCT03338790[191]	Nivolumab in combination with rucaparib, docetaxel, or enzalutamide	Phase II	Metastatic CRPC	Nivolumab blocks cancer cells' protective proteins against T cells.

(continued on next page)

Table 1
(continued)

Trial Number	Drug	Phase	Tumor Type	Mechanism of Action
NCT02601014[192]	Nivolumab and ipilimumab	Phase II	Metastatic CRPC	Ipilimumab turns off cancer mediated T-cell inhibition.
NCT03217747[193]	Avelumab, utomilumab, anti-OX40 antibody PF-04518600, and radiation therapy	Phase I/II	Metastatic CRPC	Utomilumab targets (CD137) to stimulate a more intense immune system attack on cancers.

Abbreviation: TGF, transforming growth factor.

Radiotherapy induced tumor growth delay in TRAMP-C1 prostate cancer model, but increased macrophages and dendritic cells and also causes upregulation of PD-1/PD-L1, CD8$^+$ T cells.[186] TRAMP-C1P3 cells have been derived from TRAMP-C1 and showed tumorigenic and metastatic to lymph nodes. It was demonstrated that Fms-like tyrosine kinase-3 ligand induced inflammatory cell infiltrate, including dendritic cells, macrophages, granulocytes and CD4$^+$ and CD8$^+$ T cells, significantly inhibited the growth of preexisting orthotopic TRAMP-C1P3 tumors and also the development of metastatic disease.[187]

IL-15 combination with CTLA-4 and PD-L1 blockade increased CD8$^+$ T cells, increased antitumor activity, suppressed tumor growth and prolonged the animal survival in a TRAMP-C2 prostate tumor model.[188] Imiquimod was showed to enhance antitumor activation of CD8$^+$ T cells, and imiquimod inhibits TRAMP-C2 cells in vivo and in vitro.[189,190] Enhanced IL-15Ralpha expression increased the CD8$^+$ T cells in TRAMP-C2 tumors, which resulted in inhibition of tumor growth.[191]

Syngeneic mouse models
Syngeneic mouse models, such as C57BL/6, BALB/C and FVB mice, are widely used preclinical models to study anticancer therapeutics. These models are immunocompetent and useful for testing immunotherapeutic agents. Carcinogens have been used to induce tumor formation in various strains of mice allowing researchers to understand and measure subsequent immune response and antitumor activity. This carcinogen-induced model presents a relatively useful level of genomic instability that warrants investigation of antitumor response.[192] Furthermore, genetic manipulation of the syngeneic model allows for the analysis of the effects of various biomarkers involving sensitivity or resistance responses.[193] It is very clear that owing to the ease of using these models and also because of high reproducibility, they are most commonly used preclinical models to test immunotherapies. However, these models lack the microenvironment and also the genomic heterogeneity seen in human cancer. Owing to the limited number of mice strains that researchers work with, there is a lack of interpatient genomic heterogeneity. Also, normal progression that defines the cancer growth in these models does not adequately represent the intrapatient genetic heterogeneity seen in normal individuals with metastatic prostate cancer. This posits a challenge for modeling the effects of cancer immunotherapy.[194] The other caveat is that in these syngeneic mice the implanted tumors are poorly differentiated and do not recapitulate the tumor evolution seen in human beings. Thus, the typical plasticity of the tumor evolution as well as the adaptability of the immune editing response by typical human beings is overtly absent in the syngeneic mouse models.[195] Finally, a crucial component of cancer development encompasses the surroundings microenvironment that can both facilitate and inhibit to tumor growth. Various tissue elements such as the microvasculature and stem cell progenitor populations naturally respond and adapt to tumor growth. However, these molecular components are largely absent in the subcutaneous implantation sites located in syngeneic models.[196]

Genetically engineered mouse models
A better understanding of the genetic subclasses of cancer have led to invention of genetically engineered mouse models having the specific genetic alterations incorporated and tissue specific tumor development. Tissue-specific promoters are predominantly used for driving either the expression of an oncogene or expression of recombinase

enzymes that drive the deletion of tumor suppressors. Viral oncogenes such as SV40 large T antigen,[197] or Kras and MYC[198] and so on, and tumor suppressors like PTEN and TP53 in prostate caner,[199] APC in colon cancer,[200] among others, are modeled. These models help in developing autochthonous cancer development and also the precancerous lesions such as intraepithelial neoplasia in the prostate.[201] Most important, targeting tissue specific promoters that alter the expression of normal tumor suppressor activity as well as oncogenic function engenders a long window for tumor development. Thus, there is ample time for immunotherapeutic intervention of gradual and adaptive immune responses.[202] Mimicking the complexity of oncogenesis and tumor burden seen in human patients is a goal with genetically engineered mouse models. It is important to consider the effects that increased mutational rates have on the immune system. Genetically altering tissue-specific genes leads to this increase mutational response, thus promoting the formation and existence of neoantigens. Neoantigens are recognized by cytotoxic T cells for targeted tumor destruction, which can provide helpful clues as to how to develop immunotherapeutic vaccines.[202]

Studies in mouse models could potentially aid in clinical trial design and expected outcome. One of the mouse models that has been widely studied to determine immunologic response in the TRAMP model (transgenic adenocarcinoma of the mouse prostate model).

Patient-derived xenograft

Human xenograft models are one of the oldest models for evaluating cytotoxic therapies against cancer. These models have priory advantage in the evaluation of antitumor efficacy. The hosts include athymic nude or severe combined immunodeficiency (SCID) animals.[203]

Athymic nude mice have neutrophils and dendritic cells, B cells, and natural killer cells, many aspects of the immune response, although they lack normal thymic development and are deficient in T-cell function. SCID mice lack a DNA-dependent protein kinase, which is essential for T-cell and B-cell development. Therefore, athymic nude mice were good for engraftment of human cancer cell lines, whereas the NOD/SCID mice are sufficient for engraftment of primary human tumors.[204,205] NOD/SCID mice demonstrated PD-1 targeted immunotherapy inhibited both cell line–derived xenograft and patient-derived xenograft tumor growth, indicating an important preclinical immunotherapy model for research.[206]

Humanized tumor models

Humanized tumor models depart from the previous models in the sense that they are the most relevant and representative of the cancer growth in humans. Various humanized mice models are available including humanized CD34$^+$ mouse models, humanized PBMC mouse models, and knock-in humanized mouse models.[207] These models are vital in the study of immune responses because they use patient derived xenografts, which contained human tumor tissue. The human tumor tissue is implanted into these mice models that exhibit an intact humanized immune system. They resemble human tissue in the sense that they accurately create the complexity associated with genetic heterogeneity as well as the tissue microenvironment.[208] In the humanized CD34$^+$ mouse model, the mice are initially irradiated to destroy the host immune system. Subsequently, they are injected or reconstituted with umbilical cord human CD34$^+$ cells. The development of the human immune system is monitored over 12 to 15 weeks and then the effects of the immune response to engrafted human patient-derived xenograft tumor is analyzed.[209] Recent studies have shown the efficacy of the CD34$^+$ humanized mice and positive antitumor responses in the regression of human tumor xenograft.[206] Another model, the humanized PBMC mouse models, is usually performed owing to its very short-term and robust reaction. This mouse model can be used in immunocompromised mice, to reconstitute the human immune system using peripheral blood mononuclear cells. Subcutaneous or orthotopic implantation of patient-derived xenograft or cell line derived xenograft can then be used to assess antitumor response. One of the problems with this model is that it involves a quick engraftment, which limits the time for observation of T-cell immune modulation, as well as overall antitumor activity.[210]

FUTURE DIRECTIONS: COMBINATION THERAPY OF VACCINES AND CHECKPOINT INHIBITORS, WITH MOLECULARLY DRIVEN APPROACHES

The introduction of immunotherapy to cancer treatment has brought a revolutionary change in the treatment for patients with cancer. As results of studies involving single agent immunotherapies for prostate cancer are coming out, there is a clear need for combinatorial approaches to evoke immune responses in patients with prostate cancer. Currently, there are numerous clinical trials of combined immunotherapy that are ongoing for prostate cancer. As we start to see the results from these studies as well as new therapeutics, we will learn novel methods to improve the benefits from immunotherapies for prostate cancer.

Future research directions of prostate cancer immunotherapy are mainly focus on identifying molecular mechanism of immune resistance and developing combination therapies. To develop beneficial combination immunotherapies that show promising clinical outcomes, it is important to investigate their efficacy using complex mouse models. The humanized tumor models can prove to be useful because they are used in the study of immune responses that use patient derived xenografts, which contain human tumor tissue. Mimicking the complexity of the human tumor tissue, genetic heterogeneity, and microenvironment through these mouse models, is a vital step in improved treatment outcomes. Personalized therapies combining genomically targeted therapies (gene and cell therapies), with approaches to alleviate immune response is the future direction for metastatic diseases.

ACKNOWLEDGEMENTS

The authors wish to thank Dr. Avery Davis, Department of Urology, Icahn School of Medicine at Mount Sinai, New York, New York, USA, for help with the figure of this manuscript. The authors wish to acknowledge funding support from The Arthur M. Blank Family Foundation to AT. The Figure, either in part or whole, was exported under paid subscription and created with Biorender.com.

DISCLOSURE

No competing financial and/or non-financial interests.

REFERENCES

1. Siegel RL, Miller KD, Jemal A. Cancer statistics, 2020. CA Cancer J Clin 2020;70:7–30. https://doi.org/10.3322/caac.21590.
2. Culp MB, Soerjomataram I, Efstathiou JA, et al. Recent global patterns in prostate cancer incidence and mortality rates. Eur Urol 2020;77:38–52. https://doi.org/10.1016/j.eururo.2019.08.005.
3. Baig FA, Hamid A, Mirza T, et al. Ductal and acinar adenocarcinoma of prostate: morphological and immunohistochemical characterization. Oman Med J 2015;30:162–6. https://doi.org/10.5001/omj.2015.36.
4. Miyoshi Y, Uemura H, Kitami K, et al. Neuroendocrine differentiated small cell carcinoma presenting as recurrent prostate cancer after androgen deprivation therapy. BJU Int 2001;88:982–3. https://doi.org/10.1046/j.1464-4096.2001.00936.x.
5. Shah RB, Mehra R, Chinnaiyan AM, et al. Androgen-independent prostate cancer is a heterogeneous group of diseases: lessons from a rapid autopsy program. Cancer Res 2004;64:9209–16. https://doi.org/10.1158/0008-5472.CAN-04-2442.
6. Tanaka M, Suzuki Y, Takaoka K, et al. Progression of prostate cancer to neuroendocrine cell tumor. Int J Urol 2001;8:431–6. https://doi.org/10.1046/j.1442-2042.2001.00347.x [discussion: 437].
7. Turbat-Herrera EA, Herrera GA, Gore I, et al. Neuroendocrine differentiation in prostatic carcinomas. A retrospective autopsy study. Arch Pathol Lab Med 1988;112:1100–5.
8. Cancer Genome Atlas Research Network. The molecular taxonomy of primary prostate cancer. Cell 2015;163:1011–25. https://doi.org/10.1016/j.cell.2015.10.025.
9. Taylor BS, Schultz N, Hieronymus H, et al. Integrative genomic profiling of human prostate cancer. Cancer Cell 2010;18:11–22. https://doi.org/10.1016/j.ccr.2010.05.026.
10. Tomlins SA, Bjartell A, Chinnaiyan AM, et al. ETS gene fusions in prostate cancer: from discovery to daily clinical practice. Eur Urol 2009;56:275–86. https://doi.org/10.1016/j.eururo.2009.04.036.
11. Tomlins SA, Rhodes DR, Perner S, et al. Recurrent fusion of TMPRSS2 and ETS transcription factor genes in prostate cancer. Science 2005;310:644–8. https://doi.org/10.1126/science.1117679.
12. Barbieri CE, Baca SC, Lawrence MS, et al. Exome sequencing identifies recurrent SPOP, FOXA1 and MED12 mutations in prostate cancer. Nat Genet 2012;44:685–9. https://doi.org/10.1038/ng.2279.
13. Gasi Tandefelt D, Boormans J, Hermans K, et al. ETS fusion genes in prostate cancer. Endocr Relat Cancer 2014;21:R143–52. https://doi.org/10.1530/ERC-13-0390.
14. Nam RK, Sugar L, Yang W, et al. Expression of the TMPRSS2:ERG fusion gene predicts cancer recurrence after surgery for localised prostate cancer. Br J Cancer 2007;97:1690–5. https://doi.org/10.1038/sj.bjc.6604054.
15. Geng C, He B, Xu L, et al. Prostate cancer-associated mutations in speckle-type POZ protein (SPOP) regulate steroid receptor coactivator 3 protein turnover. Proc Natl Acad Sci U S A 2013;110:6997–7002. https://doi.org/10.1073/pnas.1304502110.
16. Yoshimoto M, Cunha IW, Coudry RA, et al. FISH analysis of 107 prostate cancers shows that PTEN genomic deletion is associated with poor clinical outcome. Br J Cancer 2007;97:678–85. https://doi.org/10.1038/sj.bjc.6603924.

17. Robinson D, Van Allen EM, Wu YM, et al. Integrative clinical genomics of advanced prostate cancer. Cell 2015;162:454. https://doi.org/10.1016/j.cell.2015.06.053.

18. Ramaswamy S, Nakamura N, Vazquez F, et al. Regulation of G1 progression by the PTEN tumor suppressor protein is linked to inhibition of the phosphatidylinositol 3-kinase/Akt pathway. Proc Natl Acad Sci U S A 1999;96:2110–5. https://doi.org/10.1073/pnas.96.5.2110.

19. Shoag J, Barbieri CE. Clinical variability and molecular heterogeneity in prostate cancer. Asian J Androl 2016;18:543–8. https://doi.org/10.4103/1008-682X.178852.

20. Mu P, Zhang Z, Benelli M, et al. SOX2 promotes lineage plasticity and antiandrogen resistance in TP53- and RB1-deficient prostate cancer. Science 2017;355:84–8. https://doi.org/10.1126/science.aah4307.

21. Ku SY, Rosario S, Wang Y, et al. Rb1 and Trp53 cooperate to suppress prostate cancer lineage plasticity, metastasis, and antiandrogen resistance. Science 2017;355:78–83. https://doi.org/10.1126/science.aah4199.

22. Simmons MN, Berglund RK, Jones JS. A practical guide to prostate cancer diagnosis and management. Cleve Clin J Med 2011;78:321–31. https://doi.org/10.3949/ccjm.78a.10104.

23. Tomita N, Soga N, Ogura Y, et al. High-dose radiotherapy with helical tomotherapy and long-term androgen deprivation therapy for prostate cancer: 5-year outcomes. J Cancer Res Clin Oncol 2016; 142:1609–19. https://doi.org/10.1007/s00432-016-2173-9.

24. Preisser F, Mazzone E, Knipper S, et al. Effect of external beam radiotherapy on second primary cancer risk after radical prostatectomy. Can Urol Assoc J 2019. https://doi.org/10.5489/cuaj.6087.

25. D'Amico AV, Whittington R, Malkowicz SB, et al. Biochemical outcome after radical prostatectomy, external beam radiation therapy, or interstitial radiation therapy for clinically localized prostate cancer. JAMA 1998;280:969–74. https://doi.org/10.1001/jama.280.11.969.

26. Graefen M, Beyer B, Schlomm T. Outcome of radical prostatectomy: is it the approach or the surgical expertise? Eur Urol 2014;66:457–8. https://doi.org/10.1016/j.eururo.2013.12.010.

27. Bass R, Fleshner N, Finelli A, et al. Oncologic and functional outcomes of partial gland ablation with high intensity focused ultrasound for localized prostate cancer. J Urol 2019;201:113–9. https://doi.org/10.1016/j.juro.2018.07.040.

28. Shim M, Bang WJ, Oh CY, et al. Effectiveness of three different luteinizing hormone-releasing hormone agonists in the chemical castration of patients with prostate cancer: Goserelin versus triptorelin versus leuprolide. Investig Clin Urol 2019;60:244–50. https://doi.org/10.4111/icu.2019.60.4.244.

29. Hahn AW, Higano CS, Taplin ME, et al. Metastatic castration-sensitive prostate cancer: optimizing patient selection and treatment. Am Soc Clin Oncol Educ Book 2018;38:363–71. https://doi.org/10.1200/EDBK_200967.

30. Cornford P, Bellmunt J, Bolla M, et al. EAU-ESTRO-SIOG guidelines on prostate cancer. Part II: treatment of relapsing, metastatic, and castration-resistant prostate cancer. Eur Urol 2017;71:630–42. https://doi.org/10.1016/j.eururo.2016.08.002.

31. Lin DW, Shih MC, Aronson W, et al. Veterans Affairs Cooperative Studies Program Study #553: chemotherapy after prostatectomy for high-risk prostate carcinoma: a phase III randomized study. Eur Urol 2020;77:563–72. https://doi.org/10.1016/j.eururo.2019.12.020.

32. Cursano MC, Iuliani M, Casadei C, et al. Combination radium-223 therapies in patients with bone metastases from castration-resistant prostate cancer: a review. Crit Rev Oncol Hematol 2020;146: 102864. https://doi.org/10.1016/j.critrevonc.2020.102864.

33. Li K, Zhan W, Chen Y, et al. Docetaxel and doxorubicin codelivery by nanocarriers for synergistic treatment of prostate cancer. Front Pharmacol 2019;10:1436. https://doi.org/10.3389/fphar.2019.01436.

34. Hammer S, Hagemann UB, Zitzmann-Kolbe S, et al. Preclinical efficacy of a PSMA-targeted thorium-227 conjugate (PSMA-TTC), a targeted alpha therapy for prostate cancer. Clin Cancer Res 2019. https://doi.org/10.1158/1078-0432.CCR-19-2268.

35. DeWeerdt S. Bacteriology: a caring culture. Nature 2013;504:S4–5. https://doi.org/10.1038/504S4a.

36. Klener P Jr, Otahal P, Lateckova L, et al. Immunotherapy approaches in cancer treatment. Curr Pharm Biotechnol 2015;16:771–81. https://doi.org/10.2174/1389201016666150619114554.

37. Burnet FM. Immunological aspects of malignant disease. Lancet 1967;1:1171–4. https://doi.org/10.1016/s0140-6736(67)92837-1.

38. Smyth MJ, Godfrey DI, Trapani JA. A fresh look at tumor immunosurveillance and immunotherapy. Nat Immunol 2001;2:293–9. https://doi.org/10.1038/86297.

39. Romero P, Valmori D, Pittet MJ, et al. Antigenicity and immunogenicity of Melan-A/MART-1 derived peptides as targets for tumor reactive CTL in human melanoma. Immunol Rev 2002;188:81–96. https://doi.org/10.1034/j.1600-065x.2002.18808.x.

40. Kaplan DH, Shankaran V, Dighe AS, et al. Demonstration of an interferon gamma-dependent tumor surveillance system in immunocompetent mice.

Proc Natl Acad Sci U S A 1998;95:7556–61. https://doi.org/10.1073/pnas.95.13.7556.

41. Rosenberg SA, Yang JC, Sherry RM, et al. Durable complete responses in heavily pretreated patients with metastatic melanoma using T-cell transfer immunotherapy. Clin Cancer Res 2011;17:4550–7. https://doi.org/10.1158/1078-0432.CCR-11-0116.

42. Rosenberg SA, Lotze MT, Muul LM, et al. Observations on the systemic administration of autologous lymphokine-activated killer cells and recombinant interleukin-2 to patients with metastatic cancer. N Engl J Med 1985;313:1485–92. https://doi.org/10.1056/NEJM198512053132327.

43. Atkins MB, Lotze MT, Dutcher JP, et al. High-dose recombinant interleukin 2 therapy for patients with metastatic melanoma: analysis of 270 patients treated between 1985 and 1993. J Clin Oncol 1999;17:2105–16. https://doi.org/10.1200/JCO.1999.17.7.2105.

44. Kohler G, Milstein C. Continuous cultures of fused cells secreting antibody of predefined specificity. Nature 1975;256:495–7. https://doi.org/10.1038/256495a0.

45. Maloney DG, Grillo-Lopez AJ, White CA, et al. IDEC-C2B8 (Rituximab) anti-CD20 monoclonal antibody therapy in patients with relapsed low-grade non-Hodgkin's lymphoma. Blood 1997;90:2188–95.

46. Reff ME, Carner K, Chambers KS, et al. Depletion of B cells in vivo by a chimeric mouse human monoclonal antibody to CD20. Blood 1994;83:435–45.

47. Eshhar Z, Waks T, Gross G, et al. Specific activation and targeting of cytotoxic lymphocytes through chimeric single chains consisting of antibody-binding domains and the gamma or zeta subunits of the immunoglobulin and T-cell receptors. Proc Natl Acad Sci U S A 1993;90:720–4. https://doi.org/10.1073/pnas.90.2.720.

48. Kochenderfer JN, Wilson WH, Janik JE, et al. Eradication of B-lineage cells and regression of lymphoma in a patient treated with autologous T cells genetically engineered to recognize CD19. Blood 2010;116:4099–102. https://doi.org/10.1182/blood-2010-04-281931.

49. Brentjens RJ, Riviere I, Park JH, et al. Safety and persistence of adoptively transferred autologous CD19-targeted T cells in patients with relapsed or chemotherapy refractory B-cell leukemias. Blood 2011;118:4817–28. https://doi.org/10.1182/blood-2011-04-348540.

50. Grupp SA, Kalos M, Barrett D, et al. Chimeric antigen receptor-modified T cells for acute lymphoid leukemia. N Engl J Med 2013;368:1509–18. https://doi.org/10.1056/NEJMoa1215134.

51. Maude SL, Frey N, Shaw PA, et al. Chimeric antigen receptor T cells for sustained remissions in leukemia. N Engl J Med 2014;371:1507–17. https://doi.org/10.1056/NEJMoa1407222.

52. Schuster SJ, Svoboda J, Chong EA, et al. Chimeric antigen receptor T cells in refractory B-cell lymphomas. N Engl J Med 2017;377:2545–54. https://doi.org/10.1056/NEJMoa1708566.

53. Pehlivan KC, Duncan BB, Lee DW. CAR-T cell therapy for acute lymphoblastic leukemia: transforming the treatment of relapsed and refractory disease. Curr Hematol Malig Rep 2018;13:396–406. https://doi.org/10.1007/s11899-018-0470-x.

54. Locke FL, Neelapu SS, Bartlett NL, et al. Phase 1 results of ZUMA-1: a multicenter study of KTE-C19 Anti-CD19 CAR T cell therapy in refractory aggressive lymphoma. Mol Ther 2017;25:285–95. https://doi.org/10.1016/j.ymthe.2016.10.020.

55. McGranahan N, Furness AJ, Rosenthal R, et al. Clonal neoantigens elicit T cell immunoreactivity and sensitivity to immune checkpoint blockade. Science 2016;351:1463–9. https://doi.org/10.1126/science.aaf1490.

56. Van Allen EM, Miao D, Schilling B, et al. Genomic correlates of response to CTLA-4 blockade in metastatic melanoma. Science 2015;350:207–11. https://doi.org/10.1126/science.aad0095.

57. Snyder A, Makarov V, Merghoub T, et al. Genetic basis for clinical response to CTLA-4 blockade in melanoma. N Engl J Med 2014;371:2189–99. https://doi.org/10.1056/NEJMoa1406498.

58. van Rooij N, van Buuren MM, Philips D, et al. Tumor exome analysis reveals neoantigen-specific T-cell reactivity in an ipilimumab-responsive melanoma. J Clin Oncol 2013;31:e439–42. https://doi.org/10.1200/JCO.2012.47.7521.

59. Le DT, Durham JN, Smith KN, et al. Mismatch repair deficiency predicts response of solid tumors to PD-1 blockade. Science 2017;357:409–13. https://doi.org/10.1126/science.aan6733.

60. Domingo E, Freeman-Mills L, Rayner E, et al. Somatic POLE proofreading domain mutation, immune response, and prognosis in colorectal cancer: a retrospective, pooled biomarker study. Lancet Gastroenterol Hepatol 2016;1:207–16. https://doi.org/10.1016/S2468-1253(16)30014-0.

61. Eggink FA, Van Gool IC, Leary A, et al. Immunological profiling of molecularly classified high-risk endometrial cancers identifies POLE-mutant and microsatellite unstable carcinomas as candidates for checkpoint inhibition. Oncoimmunology 2017;6:e1264565. https://doi.org/10.1080/2162402X.2016.1264565.

62. Lim HW, Hillsamer P, Banham AH, et al. Cutting edge: direct suppression of B cells by CD4+ CD25+ regulatory T cells. J Immunol 2005;175:4180–3. https://doi.org/10.4049/jimmunol.175.7.4180.

63. Iikuni N, Lourenco EV, Hahn BH, et al. Cutting edge: regulatory T cells directly suppress B cells in systemic lupus erythematosus. J Immunol

2009;183:1518–22. https://doi.org/10.4049/jimmunol.0901163.

64. Xu A, Liu Y, Chen W, et al. TGF-beta-induced regulatory T cells directly suppress B cell responses through a noncytotoxic mechanism. J Immunol 2016;196:3631–41. https://doi.org/10.4049/jimmunol.1501740.

65. Zhao DM, Thornton AM, DiPaolo RJ, et al. Activated CD4+CD25+ T cells selectively kill B lymphocytes. Blood 2006;107:3925–32. https://doi.org/10.1182/blood-2005-11-4502.

66. Bray F, Ferlay J, Soerjomataram I, et al. Global cancer statistics 2018: GLOBOCAN estimates of incidence and mortality worldwide for 36 cancers in 185 countries. CA Cancer J Clin 2018;68:394–424. https://doi.org/10.3322/caac.21492.

67. Moch H, Cubilla AL, Humphrey PA, et al. The 2016 WHO classification of tumours of the urinary system and male genital organs-part A: renal, penile, and testicular tumours. Eur Urol 2016;70:93–105. https://doi.org/10.1016/j.eururo.2016.02.029.

68. Noessner E, Brech D, Mendler AN, et al. Intratumoral alterations of dendritic-cell differentiation and CD8(+) T-cell anergy are immune escape mechanisms of clear cell renal cell carcinoma. Oncoimmunology 2012;1:1451–3. https://doi.org/10.4161/onci.21356.

69. Itsumi M, Tatsugami K. Immunotherapy for renal cell carcinoma. Clin Dev Immunol 2010;2010:284581. https://doi.org/10.1155/2010/284581.

70. Minasian LM, Motzer RJ, Gluck L, et al. Interferon alfa-2a in advanced renal cell carcinoma: treatment results and survival in 159 patients with long-term follow-up. J Clin Oncol 1993;11:1368–75. https://doi.org/10.1200/JCO.1993.11.7.1368.

71. Fyfe G, Fisher RI, Rosenberg SA, et al. Results of treatment of 255 patients with metastatic renal cell carcinoma who received high-dose recombinant interleukin-2 therapy. J Clin Oncol 1995;13:688–96. https://doi.org/10.1200/JCO.1995.13.3.688.

72. McDermott DF, Regan MM, Clark JI, et al. Randomized phase III trial of high-dose interleukin-2 versus subcutaneous interleukin-2 and interferon in patients with metastatic renal cell carcinoma. J Clin Oncol 2005;23:133–41. https://doi.org/10.1200/JCO.2005.03.206.

73. Topalian SL, Drake CG, Pardoll DM. Immune checkpoint blockade: a common denominator approach to cancer therapy. Cancer Cell 2015;27:450–61. https://doi.org/10.1016/j.ccell.2015.03.001.

74. Yang JC, Hughes M, Kammula U, et al. Ipilimumab (anti-CTLA4 antibody) causes regression of metastatic renal cell cancer associated with enteritis and hypophysitis. J Immunother 2007;30:825–30. https://doi.org/10.1097/CJI.0b013e318156e47e.

75. Topalian SL, Hodi FS, Brahmer JR, et al. Safety, activity, and immune correlates of anti-PD-1 antibody in cancer. N Engl J Med 2012;366:2443–54. https://doi.org/10.1056/NEJMoa1200690.

76. Wallin JJ, Bendell JC, Funke R, et al. Atezolizumab in combination with bevacizumab enhances antigen-specific T-cell migration in metastatic renal cell carcinoma. Nat Commun 2016;7:12624. https://doi.org/10.1038/ncomms12624.

77. Elamin YY, Rafee S, Toomey S, et al. Immune effects of bevacizumab: killing two birds with one stone. Cancer Microenviron 2015;8:15–21. https://doi.org/10.1007/s12307-014-0160-8.

78. McDermott DF, Huseni MA, Atkins MB, et al. Clinical activity and molecular correlates of response to atezolizumab alone or in combination with bevacizumab versus sunitinib in renal cell carcinoma. Nat Med 2018;24:749–57. https://doi.org/10.1038/s41591-018-0053-3.

79. Rini BI, Powles T, Atkins MB, et al. Atezolizumab plus bevacizumab versus sunitinib in patients with previously untreated metastatic renal cell carcinoma (IMmotion151): a multicentre, open-label, phase 3, randomised controlled trial. Lancet 2019;393:2404–15. https://doi.org/10.1016/S0140-6736(19)30723-8.

80. Motzer RJ, Penkov K, Haanen J, et al. Avelumab plus axitinib versus sunitinib for advanced renal-cell carcinoma. N Engl J Med 2019;380:1103–15. https://doi.org/10.1056/NEJMoa1816047.

81. Atkins MB, Plimack ER, Puzanov I, et al. Axitinib in combination with pembrolizumab in patients with advanced renal cell cancer: a non-randomised, open-label, dose-finding, and dose-expansion phase 1b trial. Lancet Oncol 2018;19:405–15. https://doi.org/10.1016/S1470-2045(18)30081-0.

82. Rini BI, Plimack ER, Stus V, et al. Pembrolizumab plus axitinib versus sunitinib for advanced renal-cell carcinoma. N Engl J Med 2019;380:1116–27. https://doi.org/10.1056/NEJMoa1816714.

83. Shelley MD, Kynaston H, Court J, et al. A systematic review of intravesical bacillus Calmette-Guerin plus transurethral resection vs transurethral resection alone in Ta and T1 bladder cancer. BJU Int 2001;88:209–16. https://doi.org/10.1046/j.1464-410x.2001.02306.x.

84. Bohle A, Jocham D, Bock PR. Intravesical bacillus Calmette-Guerin versus mitomycin C for superficial bladder cancer: a formal meta-analysis of comparative studies on recurrence and toxicity. J Urol 2003;169:90–5. https://doi.org/10.1097/01.ju.0000039680.90768.b3.

85. Morales A, Eidinger D, Bruce AW. Intracavitary Bacillus Calmette-Guerin in the treatment of superficial bladder tumors. J Urol 1976;116:180–3. https://doi.org/10.1016/s0022-5347(17)58737-6.

86. Lamm DL, Thor DE, Harris SC, et al. Bacillus Calmette-Guerin immunotherapy of superficial bladder cancer. J Urol 1980;124:38–40. https://doi.org/10.1016/s0022-5347(17)55282-9.

87. Lamm DL, Thor DE, Stogdill VD, et al. Bladder cancer immunotherapy. J Urol 1982;128:931–5. https://doi.org/10.1016/s0022-5347(17)53283-8.

88. Brosman SA. Experience with bacillus Calmette-Guerin in patients with superficial bladder carcinoma. J Urol 1982;128:27–30. https://doi.org/10.1016/s0022-5347(17)52736-6.

89. Schellhammer PF, Ladaga LE, Fillion MB. Bacillus Calmette-Guerin for superficial transitional cell carcinoma of the bladder. J Urol 1986;135:261–4. https://doi.org/10.1016/s0022-5347(17)45603-5.

90. Martinez-Pineiro JA, Jimenez Leon J, Martinez-Pineiro L, et al. Bacillus Calmette-Guerin versus doxorubicin versus thiotepa: a randomized prospective study in 202 patients with superficial bladder cancer. J Urol 1990;143:502–6. https://doi.org/10.1016/s0022-5347(17)40002-4.

91. Lamm DL, Blumenstein BA, Crawford ED, et al. A randomized trial of intravesical doxorubicin and immunotherapy with bacille Calmette-Guerin for transitional-cell carcinoma of the bladder. N Engl J Med 1991;325:1205–9. https://doi.org/10.1056/NEJM199110243251703.

92. Witjes JA. Management of BCG failures in superficial bladder cancer: a review. Eur Urol 2006;49:790–7. https://doi.org/10.1016/j.eururo.2006.01.017.

93. Rosenberg JE, Hoffman-Censits J, Powles T, et al. Atezolizumab in patients with locally advanced and metastatic urothelial carcinoma who have progressed following treatment with platinum-based chemotherapy: a single-arm, multicentre, phase 2 trial. Lancet 2016;387:1909–20. https://doi.org/10.1016/S0140-6736(16)00561-4.

94. Powles T, O'Donnell PH, Massard C, et al. Efficacy and safety of durvalumab in locally advanced or metastatic urothelial carcinoma: updated results from a phase 1/2 open-label study. JAMA Oncol 2017;3:e172411. https://doi.org/10.1001/jamaoncol.2017.2411.

95. Apolo AB, Infante JR, Balmanoukian A, et al. Avelumab, an anti-programmed death-ligand 1 antibody, in patients with refractory metastatic urothelial carcinoma: results from a multicenter, phase Ib study. J Clin Oncol 2017;35:2117–24. https://doi.org/10.1200/JCO.2016.71.6795.

96. Sharma P, Retz M, Siefker-Radtke A, et al. Nivolumab in metastatic urothelial carcinoma after platinum therapy (CheckMate 275): a multicentre, single-arm, phase 2 trial. Lancet Oncol 2017;18:312–22. https://doi.org/10.1016/S1470-2045(17)30065-7.

97. Bellmunt J, Bajorin DF. Pembrolizumab for advanced urothelial carcinoma. N Engl J Med 2017;376:2304. https://doi.org/10.1056/NEJMc1704612.

98. Powles T, Eder JP, Fine GD, et al. MPDL3280A (anti-PD-L1) treatment leads to clinical activity in metastatic bladder cancer. Nature 2014;515:558–62. https://doi.org/10.1038/nature13904.

99. Necchi A, Joseph RW, Loriot Y, et al. Atezolizumab in platinum-treated locally advanced or metastatic urothelial carcinoma: post-progression outcomes from the phase II IMvigor210 study. Ann Oncol 2017;28:3044–50. https://doi.org/10.1093/annonc/mdx518.

100. Sharma P, Callahan MK, Bono P, et al. Nivolumab monotherapy in recurrent metastatic urothelial carcinoma (CheckMate 032): a multicentre, open-label, two-stage, multi-arm, phase 1/2 trial. Lancet Oncol 2016;17:1590–8. https://doi.org/10.1016/S1470-2045(16)30496-X.

101. Ohyama C, Kojima T, Kondo T, et al. Nivolumab in patients with unresectable locally advanced or metastatic urothelial carcinoma: CheckMate 275 2-year global and Japanese patient population analyses. Int J Clin Oncol 2019;24:1089–98. https://doi.org/10.1007/s10147-019-01450-w.

102. Bellmunt J, de Wit R, Vaughn DJ, et al. Pembrolizumab as second-line therapy for advanced urothelial carcinoma. N Engl J Med 2017;376:1015–26. https://doi.org/10.1056/NEJMoa1613683.

103. Hanna NH, Einhorn LH. Testicular cancer–discoveries and updates. N Engl J Med 2014;371:2005–16. https://doi.org/10.1056/NEJMra1407550.

104. Galvez-Carvajal L, Sanchez-Munoz A, Ribelles N, et al. Targeted treatment approaches in refractory germ cell tumors. Crit Rev Oncol Hematol 2019;143:130–8. https://doi.org/10.1016/j.critrevonc.2019.09.005.

105. Menk AV, Scharping NE, Rivadeneira DB, et al. 4-1BB costimulation induces T cell mitochondrial function and biogenesis enabling cancer immunotherapeutic responses. J Exp Med 2018;215:1091–100. https://doi.org/10.1084/jem.20171068.

106. Danaher P, Warren S, Lu R, et al. Pan-cancer adaptive immune resistance as defined by the tumor inflammation signature (TIS): results from the Cancer Genome Atlas (TCGA). J Immunother Cancer 2018;6:63. https://doi.org/10.1186/s40425-018-0367-1.

107. Kiniwa Y, Miyahara Y, Wang HY, et al. CD8+ Foxp3+ regulatory T cells mediate immunosuppression in prostate cancer. Clin Cancer Res 2007;13:6947–58. https://doi.org/10.1158/1078-0432.CCR-07-0842.

108. Kaur HB, Guedes LB, Lu J, et al. Association of tumor-infiltrating T-cell density with molecular subtype, racial ancestry and clinical outcomes in prostate cancer. Mod Pathol 2018;31:1539–52. https://doi.org/10.1038/s41379-018-0083-x.

109. Nardone V, Botta C, Caraglia M, et al. Tumor infiltrating T lymphocytes expressing FoxP3, CCR7 or PD-1 predict the outcome of prostate cancer patients subjected to salvage radiotherapy after biochemical relapse. Cancer Biol Ther 2016;17:1213–20. https://doi.org/10.1080/15384047.2016.1235666.

110. Lundholm M, Hagglof C, Wikberg ML, et al. Secreted factors from colorectal and prostate cancer cells skew the immune response in opposite directions. Sci Rep 2015;5:15651. https://doi.org/10.1038/srep15651.

111. Mariathasan S, Turley SJ, Nickles D, et al. TGFbeta attenuates tumour response to PD-L1 blockade by contributing to exclusion of T cells. Nature 2018;554:544–8. https://doi.org/10.1038/nature25501.

112. Lawrence MS, Stojanov P, Polak P, et al. Mutational heterogeneity in cancer and the search for new cancer-associated genes. Nature 2013;499:214–8. https://doi.org/10.1038/nature12213.

113. Freedland SJ, Aronson WJ. Commentary on "Integrative clinical genomics of advanced prostate cancer". Robinson D, Van Allen EM, Wu YM, Schultz N, Lonigro RJ, Mosquera JM, Montgomery B, Taplin ME, Pritchard CC, Attard G, Beltran H, Abida W, Bradley RK, Vinson J, Cao X, Vats P, Kunju LP, Hussain M, Feng FY, Tomlins SA, Cooney KA, Smith DC, Brennan C, Siddiqui J, Mehra R, Chen Y, Rathkopf DE, Morris MJ, Solomon SB, Durack JC, Reuter VE, Gopalan A, Gao J, Loda M, Lis RT, Bowden M, Balk SP, Gaviola G, Sougnez C, Gupta M, Yu EY, Mostaghel EA, Cheng HH, Mulcahy H, True LD, Plymate SR, Dvinge H, Ferraldeschi R, Flohr P, Miranda S, Zafeiriou Z, Tunariu N, Mateo J, Perez-Lopez R, Demichelis F, Robinson BD, Schiffman M, Nanus DM, Tagawa ST, Sigaras A, Eng KW, Elemento O, Sboner A, Heath EI, Scher HI, Pienta KJ, Kantoff P, de Bono JS, Rubin MA, Nelson PS, Garraway LA, Sawyers CL, Chinnaiyan AM.Cell. 21 May 2015;161(5):1215-1228. Urol Oncol 2017;35:535. https://doi.org/10.1016/j.urolonc.2017.05.010.

114. Pritchard CC, Mateo J, Walsh MF, et al. Inherited DNA-repair gene mutations in men with metastatic prostate cancer. N Engl J Med 2016;375:443–53. https://doi.org/10.1056/NEJMoa1603144.

115. Drake CG, Lipson EJ, Brahmer JR. Breathing new life into immunotherapy: review of melanoma, lung and kidney cancer. Nat Rev Clin Oncol 2014;11:24–37. https://doi.org/10.1038/nrclinonc.2013.208.

116. Mac Keon S, Ruiz MS, Gazzaniga S, et al. Dendritic cell-based vaccination in cancer: therapeutic implications emerging from murine models. Front Immunol 2015;6:243. https://doi.org/10.3389/fimmu.2015.00243.

117. Westdorp H, Skold AE, Snijer BA, et al. Immunotherapy for prostate cancer: lessons from responses to tumor-associated antigens. Front Immunol 2014;5:191. https://doi.org/10.3389/fimmu.2014.00191.

118. Kantoff PW, Higano CS, Shore ND, et al. Sipuleucel-T immunotherapy for castration-resistant prostate cancer. N Engl J Med 2010;363:411–22. https://doi.org/10.1056/NEJMoa1001294.

119. Ren R, Koti M, Hamilton T, et al. A primer on tumour immunology and prostate cancer immunotherapy. Can Urol Assoc J 2016;10:60–5. https://doi.org/10.5489/cuaj.3418.

120. Gilboa E. DC-based cancer vaccines. J Clin Invest 2007;117:1195–203. https://doi.org/10.1172/JCI31205.

121. Drake CG. Prostate cancer as a model for tumour immunotherapy. Nat Rev Immunol 2010;10:580–93. https://doi.org/10.1038/nri2817.

122. Harzstark AL, Small EJ. Immunotherapy for prostate cancer using antigen-loaded antigen-presenting cells: APC8015 (Provenge). Expert Opin Biol Ther 2007;7:1275–80. https://doi.org/10.1517/14712598.7.8.1275.

123. Simons JW, Sacks N. Granulocyte-macrophage colony-stimulating factor-transduced allogeneic cancer cellular immunotherapy: the GVAX vaccine for prostate cancer. Urol Oncol 2006;24:419–24. https://doi.org/10.1016/j.urolonc.2005.08.021.

124. Small EJ, Sacks N, Nemunaitis J, et al. Granulocyte macrophage colony-stimulating factor–secreting allogeneic cellular immunotherapy for hormone-refractory prostate cancer. Clin Cancer Res 2007;13:3883–91. https://doi.org/10.1158/1078-0432.CCR-06-2937.

125. Higano CS, Corman JM, Smith DC, et al. Phase 1/2 dose-escalation study of a GM-CSF-secreting, allogeneic, cellular immunotherapy for metastatic hormone-refractory prostate cancer. Cancer 2008;113:975–84. https://doi.org/10.1002/cncr.23669.

126. Fernandez-Garcia EM, Vera-Badillo FE, Perez-Valderrama B, et al. Immunotherapy in prostate cancer: review of the current evidence. Clin Transl Oncol 2015;17:339–57. https://doi.org/10.1007/s12094-014-1259-6.

127. Madan RA, Arlen PM, Mohebtash M, et al. Prostvac-VF: a vector-based vaccine targeting PSA in prostate cancer. Expert Opin Investig Drugs 2009;18:1001–11. https://doi.org/10.1517/13543780902997928.

128. DiPaola RS, Chen YH, Bubley GJ, et al. A national multicenter phase 2 study of prostate-specific antigen (PSA) pox virus vaccine with sequential androgen ablation therapy in patients with PSA progression: ECOG 9802. Eur Urol 2015;68:365–71. https://doi.org/10.1016/j.eururo.2014.12.010.

129. Kantoff PW, Schuetz TJ, Blumenstein BA, et al. Overall survival analysis of a phase II randomized controlled trial of a Poxviral-based PSA-targeted immunotherapy in metastatic castration-resistant prostate cancer. J Clin Oncol 2010;28:1099–105. https://doi.org/10.1200/JCO.2009.25.0597.

130. Gulley JL, Borre M, Vogelzang NJ, et al. Phase III Trial of PROSTVAC in asymptomatic or minimally symptomatic metastatic castration-resistant prostate cancer. J Clin Oncol 2019;37:1051–61. https://doi.org/10.1200/JCO.18.02031.

131. Martins KA, Bavari S, Salazar AM. Vaccine adjuvant uses of poly-IC and derivatives. Expert Rev Vaccin 2015;14:447–59. https://doi.org/10.1586/14760584.2015.966085.

132. McCartney S, Vermi W, Gilfillan S, et al. Distinct and complementary functions of MDA5 and TLR3 in poly(I:C)-mediated activation of mouse NK cells. J Exp Med 2009;206:2967–76. https://doi.org/10.1084/jem.20091181.

133. Zhang Z, Kim T, Bao M, et al. DDX1, DDX21, and DHX36 helicases form a complex with the adaptor molecule TRIF to sense dsRNA in dendritic cells. Immunity 2011;34:866–78. https://doi.org/10.1016/j.immuni.2011.03.027.

134. Lipson EJ, Drake CG. Ipilimumab: an anti-CTLA-4 antibody for metastatic melanoma. Clin Cancer Res 2011;17:6958–62. https://doi.org/10.1158/1078-0432.CCR-11-1595.

135. Egen JG, Kuhns MS, Allison JP. CTLA-4: new insights into its biological function and use in tumor immunotherapy. Nat Immunol 2002;3:611–8. https://doi.org/10.1038/ni0702-611.

136. Slovin SF, Higano CS, Hamid O, et al. Ipilimumab alone or in combination with radiotherapy in metastatic castration-resistant prostate cancer: results from an open-label, multicenter phase I/II study. Ann Oncol 2013;24:1813–21. https://doi.org/10.1093/annonc/mdt107.

137. Kwon ED, Drake CG, Scher HI, et al. Ipilimumab versus placebo after radiotherapy in patients with metastatic castration-resistant prostate cancer that had progressed after docetaxel chemotherapy (CA184-043): a multicentre, randomised, double-blind, phase 3 trial. Lancet Oncol 2014;15:700–12. https://doi.org/10.1016/S1470-2045(14)70189-5.

138. Pritchard CC, Morrissey C, Kumar A, et al. Complex MSH2 and MSH6 mutations in hypermutated microsatellite unstable advanced prostate cancer. Nat Commun 2014;5:4988. https://doi.org/10.1038/ncomms5988.

139. Antonarakis ES, Piulats JM, Gross-Goupil M, et al. Pembrolizumab for treatment-refractory metastatic castration-resistant prostate cancer: multicohort, open-label phase II KEYNOTE-199 study. J Clin Oncol 2020;38:395–405. https://doi.org/10.1200/JCO.19.01638.

140. Pembrolizumab monotherapy is active in metastatic prostate cancer. Cancer Discov 2020;10:15. https://doi.org/10.1158/2159-8290.CD-RW2019-181.

141. Boussiotis VA. Molecular and biochemical aspects of the PD-1 checkpoint pathway. N Engl J Med 2016;375:1767–78. https://doi.org/10.1056/NEJMra1514296.

142. Ahmadzadeh M, Johnson LA, Heemskerk B, et al. Tumor antigen-specific CD8 T cells infiltrating the tumor express high levels of PD-1 and are functionally impaired. Blood 2009;114:1537–44. https://doi.org/10.1182/blood-2008-12-195792.

143. Parry RV, Chemnitz JM, Frauwirth KA, et al. CTLA-4 and PD-1 receptors inhibit T-cell activation by distinct mechanisms. Mol Cell Biol 2005;25:9543–53. https://doi.org/10.1128/MCB.25.21.9543-9553.2005.

144. Goswami S, Aparicio A, Subudhi SK. Immune checkpoint therapies in prostate cancer. Cancer J 2016;22:117–20. https://doi.org/10.1097/PPO.0000000000000176.

145. McDermott DF, Atkins MB. PD-1 as a potential target in cancer therapy. Cancer Med 2013;2:662–73. https://doi.org/10.1002/cam4.106.

146. Taube JM, Klein A, Brahmer JR, et al. Association of PD-1, PD-1 ligands, and other features of the tumor immune microenvironment with response to anti-PD-1 therapy. Clin Cancer Res 2014;20:5064–74. https://doi.org/10.1158/1078-0432.CCR-13-3271.

147. Brahmer JR, Drake CG, Wollner I, et al. Phase I study of single-agent anti-programmed death-1 (MDX-1106) in refractory solid tumors: safety, clinical activity, pharmacodynamics, and immunologic correlates. J Clin Oncol 2010;28:3167–75. https://doi.org/10.1200/JCO.2009.26.7609.

148. Smith KA, Gilbride KJ, Favata MF. Lymphocyte activating factor promotes T-cell growth factor production by cloned murine lymphoma cells. Nature 1980;287:853–5. https://doi.org/10.1038/287853a0.

149. Yunger S, Bar El A, Zeltzer LA, et al. Tumor-infiltrating lymphocytes from human prostate tumors reveal anti-tumor reactivity and potential for adoptive cell therapy. Oncoimmunology 2019;8:e1672494. https://doi.org/10.1080/2162402X.2019.1672494.

150. Dannull J, Diener PA, Prikler L, et al. Prostate stem cell antigen is a promising candidate for immunotherapy of advanced prostate cancer. Cancer Res 2000;60:5522–8.

151. Kiessling A, Schmitz M, Stevanovic S, et al. Prostate stem cell antigen: identification of immunogenic peptides and assessment of reactive CD8+ T cells in prostate cancer patients. Int J Cancer 2002;102:390–7. https://doi.org/10.1002/ijc.10713.

152. Matsueda S, Kobayashi K, Nonaka Y, et al. Identification of new prostate stem cell antigen-derived peptides immunogenic in HLA-A2(+) patients with hormone-refractory prostate cancer. Cancer Immunol Immunother 2004;53:479–89. https://doi.org/10.1007/s00262-003-0464-x.

153. Garcia-Hernandez Mde L, Gray A, Hubby B, et al. Prostate stem cell antigen vaccination induces a long-term protective immune response against prostate cancer in the absence of autoimmunity. Cancer Res 2008;68:861–9. https://doi.org/10.1158/0008-5472.CAN-07-0445.

154. Krupa M, Canamero M, Gomez CE, et al. Immunization with recombinant DNA and modified vaccinia virus Ankara (MVA) vectors delivering PSCA and STEAP1 antigens inhibits prostate cancer progression. Vaccine 2011;29:1504–13. https://doi.org/10.1016/j.vaccine.2010.12.016.

155. Ross S, Spencer SD, Holcomb I, et al. Prostate stem cell antigen as therapy target: tissue expression and in vivo efficacy of an immunoconjugate. Cancer Res 2002;62:2546–53.

156. Saffran DC, Raitano AB, Hubert RS, et al. Anti-PSCA mAbs inhibit tumor growth and metastasis formation and prolong the survival of mice bearing human prostate cancer xenografts. Proc Natl Acad Sci U S A 2001;98:2658–63. https://doi.org/10.1073/pnas.051624698.

157. Olafsen T, Gu Z, Sherman MA, et al. Targeting, imaging, and therapy using a humanized antiprostate stem cell antigen (PSCA) antibody. J Immunother 2007;30:396–405. https://doi.org/10.1097/CJI.0b013e318031b53b.

158. Lu J, Celis E. Recognition of prostate tumor cells by cytotoxic T lymphocytes specific for prostate-specific membrane antigen. Cancer Res 2002;62:5807–12.

159. Harada M, Matsueda S, Yao A, et al. Prostate-related antigen-derived new peptides having the capacity of inducing prostate cancer-reactive CTLs in HLA-A2+ prostate cancer patients. Oncol Rep 2004;12:601–7.

160. Schroers R, Shen L, Rollins L, et al. Human telomerase reverse transcriptase-specific T-helper responses induced by promiscuous major histocompatibility complex class II-restricted epitopes. Clin Cancer Res 2003;9:4743–55.

161. Kobayashi H, Omiya R, Sodey B, et al. Identification of naturally processed helper T-cell epitopes from prostate-specific membrane antigen using peptide-based in vitro stimulation. Clin Cancer Res 2003;9:5386–93.

162. Zuccolotto G, Fracasso G, Merlo A, et al. PSMA-specific CAR-engineered T cells eradicate disseminated prostate cancer in preclinical models. PLoS One 2014;9:e109427. https://doi.org/10.1371/journal.pone.0109427.

163. Ma Q, Gomes EM, Lo AS, et al. Advanced generation anti-prostate specific membrane antigen designer T cells for prostate cancer immunotherapy. Prostate 2014;74:286–96. https://doi.org/10.1002/pros.22749.

164. Zhang Q, Helfand BT, Carneiro BA, et al. Efficacy against human prostate cancer by prostate-specific membrane antigen-specific, transforming growth factor-beta insensitive genetically targeted CD8(+) T-cells derived from patients with metastatic castrate-resistant disease. Eur Urol 2018;73:648–52. https://doi.org/10.1016/j.eururo.2017.12.008.

165. Lee P, Gujar S. Potentiating prostate cancer immunotherapy with oncolytic viruses. Nat Rev Urol 2018;15:235–50. https://doi.org/10.1038/nrurol.2018.10.

166. Liu GB, Zhao L, Zhang L, et al. Virus, oncolytic virus and human prostate cancer. Curr Cancer Drug Targets 2017;17:522–33. https://doi.org/10.2174/1568009616666161216095308.

167. Kohlhapp FJ, Zloza A, Kaufman HL. Talimogene laherparepvec (T-VEC) as cancer immunotherapy. Drugs Today (Barc) 2015;51:549–58. https://doi.org/10.1358/dot.2015.51.9.2383044.

168. Jhawar SR, Thandoni A, Bommareddy PK, et al. Oncolytic viruses-natural and genetically engineered cancer immunotherapies. Front Oncol 2017;7:202. https://doi.org/10.3389/fonc.2017.00202.

169. DeWeese TL, van der Poel H, Li S, et al. A phase I trial of CV706, a replication-competent, PSA selective oncolytic adenovirus, for the treatment of locally recurrent prostate cancer following radiation therapy. Cancer Res 2001;61:7464–72.

170. Mao LJ, Zhang J, Liu N, et al. Oncolytic virus carrying shRNA targeting SATB1 inhibits prostate cancer growth and metastasis. Tumour Biol 2015;36:9073–81. https://doi.org/10.1007/s13277-015-3658-x.

171. Urbiola C, Santer FR, Petersson M, et al. Oncolytic activity of the rhabdovirus VSV-GP against prostate cancer. Int J Cancer 2018;143:1786–96. https://doi.org/10.1002/ijc.31556.

172. Wustemann T, Haberkorn U, Babich J, et al. Targeting prostate cancer: prostate-specific membrane antigen based diagnosis and therapy. Med Res Rev 2019;39:40–69. https://doi.org/10.1002/med.21508.

173. Cho S, Zammarchi F, Williams DG, et al. Antitumor activity of MEDI3726 (ADCT-401), a pyrrolobenzodiazepine antibody-drug conjugate targeting PSMA, in preclinical models of prostate cancer. Mol Cancer Ther 2018;17:2176–86. https://doi.org/10.1158/1535-7163.MCT-17-0982.

174. Tanaka H, Kono E, Tran CP, et al. Monoclonal antibody targeting of N-cadherin inhibits prostate

cancer growth, metastasis and castration resistance. Nat Med 2010;16:1414–20. https://doi.org/10.1038/nm.2236.

175. Shi SJ, Wang LJ, Han DH, et al. Therapeutic effects of human monoclonal PSMA antibody-mediated TRIM24 siRNA delivery in PSMA-positive castration-resistant prostate cancer. Theranostics 2019;9:1247–63. https://doi.org/10.7150/thno.29884.

176. Waite JC, Wang B, Haber L, et al. Tumor-targeted CD28 bispecific antibodies enhance the antitumor efficacy of PD-1 immunotherapy. Sci Transl Med 2020;12. https://doi.org/10.1126/scitranslmed.aba2325.

177. Goicochea NL, Garnovskaya M, Blanton MG, et al. Development of cell-penetrating bispecific antibodies targeting the N-terminal domain of androgen receptor for prostate cancer therapy. Protein Eng Des Sel 2017;30:785–93. https://doi.org/10.1093/protein/gzx058.

178. Bailis J, Deegen P, Thomas O, et al. Preclinical evaluation of AMG 160, a next-generation bispecific T cell engager (BiTE) targeting the prostate-specific membrane antigen PSMA for metastatic castration-resistant prostate cancer (mCRPC). J Clin Oncol 2019;37:301. https://doi.org/10.1200/JCO.2019.37.7_suppl.301.

179. Thompson TC, Southgate J, Kitchener G, et al. Multistage carcinogenesis induced by ras and myc oncogenes in a reconstituted organ. Cell 1989;56:917–30. https://doi.org/10.1016/0092-8674(89)90625-9.

180. Baley PA, Yoshida K, Qian W, et al. Progression to androgen insensitivity in a novel in vitro mouse model for prostate cancer. J Steroid Biochem Mol Biol 1995;52:403–13. https://doi.org/10.1016/0960-0760(95)00001-g.

181. Yeon A, Wang Y, Su S, et al. Syngeneic murine model for prostate cancer using RM1 cells transfected with gp100. Prostate 2020;80:424–31. https://doi.org/10.1002/pros.23957.

182. Xu N, Huang L, Li X, et al. The novel combination of nitroxoline and PD-1 blockade, exerts a potent antitumor effect in a mouse model of prostate cancer. Int J Biol Sci 2019;15:919–28. https://doi.org/10.7150/ijbs.32259.

183. Foster BA, Gingrich JR, Kwon ED, et al. Characterization of prostatic epithelial cell lines derived from transgenic adenocarcinoma of the mouse prostate (TRAMP) model. Cancer Res 1997;57:3325–30.

184. Dalezis P, Geromichalos GD, Trafalis DT, et al. Dexamethasone plus octreotide regimen increases anticancer effects of docetaxel on TRAMP-C1 prostate cancer model. In Vivo 2012;26:75–86.

185. Matsumura S, Demaria S. Up-regulation of the proinflammatory chemokine CXCL16 is a common response of tumor cells to ionizing radiation. Radiat Res 2010;173:418–25. https://doi.org/10.1667/RR1860.1.

186. Philippou Y, Sjoberg HT, Murphy E, et al. Impacts of combining anti-PD-L1 immunotherapy and radiotherapy on the tumour immune microenvironment in a murine prostate cancer model. Br J Cancer 2020. https://doi.org/10.1038/s41416-020-0956-x.

187. Ciavarra RP, Holterman DA, Brown RR, et al. Prostate tumor microenvironment alters immune cells and prevents long-term survival in an orthotopic mouse model following flt3-ligand/CD40-ligand immunotherapy. J Immunother 2004;27:13–26. https://doi.org/10.1097/00002371-200401000-00002.

188. Yu P, Steel JC, Zhang M, et al. Simultaneous inhibition of two regulatory T-cell subsets enhanced Interleukin-15 efficacy in a prostate tumor model. Proc Natl Acad Sci U S A 2012;109:6187–92. https://doi.org/10.1073/pnas.1203479109.

189. Rechtsteiner G, Warger T, Osterloh P, et al. Cutting edge: priming of CTL by transcutaneous peptide immunization with imiquimod. J Immunol 2005;174:2476–80. https://doi.org/10.4049/jimmunol.174.5.2476.

190. Han JH, Lee J, Jeon SJ, et al. In vitro and in vivo growth inhibition of prostate cancer by the small molecule imiquimod. Int J Oncol 2013;42:2087–93. https://doi.org/10.3892/ijo.2013.1898.

191. Zhang M, Ju W, Yao Z, et al. Augmented IL-15Ralpha expression by CD40 activation is critical in synergistic CD8 T cell-mediated antitumor activity of anti-CD40 antibody with IL-15 in TRAMP-C2 tumors in mice. J Immunol 2012;188:6156–64. https://doi.org/10.4049/jimmunol.1102604.

192. Fantini D, Glaser AP, Rimar KJ, et al. A carcinogen-induced mouse model recapitulates the molecular alterations of human muscle invasive bladder cancer. Oncogene 2018;37:1911–25. https://doi.org/10.1038/s41388-017-0099-6.

193. Jackson SP, Bartek J. The DNA-damage response in human biology and disease. Nature 2009;461:1071–8. https://doi.org/10.1038/nature08467.

194. Salk JJ, Fox EJ, Loeb LA. Mutational heterogeneity in human cancers: origin and consequences. Annu Rev Pathol 2010;5:51–75. https://doi.org/10.1146/annurev-pathol-121808-102113.

195. Schreiber RD, Old LJ, Smyth MJ. Cancer immunoediting: integrating immunity's roles in cancer suppression and promotion. Science 2011;331:1565–70. https://doi.org/10.1126/science.1203486.

196. Bonnotte B, Gough M, Phan V, et al. Intradermal injection, as opposed to subcutaneous injection, enhances immunogenicity and suppresses tumorigenicity of tumor cells. Cancer Res 2003;63:2145–9.

197. Greenberg NM, DeMayo F, Finegold MJ, et al. Prostate cancer in a transgenic mouse. Proc Natl

Acad Sci U S A 1995;92:3439–43. https://doi.org/10.1073/pnas.92.8.3439.

198. Sinn E, Muller W, Pattengale P, et al. Coexpression of MMTV/v-Ha-ras and MMTV/c-myc genes in transgenic mice: synergistic action of oncogenes in vivo. Cell 1987;49:465–75. https://doi.org/10.1016/0092-8674(87)90449-1.

199. Chen Z, Trotman LC, Shaffer D, et al. Crucial role of p53-dependent cellular senescence in suppression of Pten-deficient tumorigenesis. Nature 2005;436:725–30. https://doi.org/10.1038/nature03918.

200. Shibata H, Toyama K, Shioya H, et al. Rapid colorectal adenoma formation initiated by conditional targeting of the Apc gene. Science 1997;278:120–3. https://doi.org/10.1126/science.278.5335.120.

201. Kaplan-Lefko PJ, Chen TM, Ittmann MM, et al. Pathobiology of autochthonous prostate cancer in a pre-clinical transgenic mouse model. Prostate 2003;55:219–37. https://doi.org/10.1002/pros.10215.

202. Liu J, Blake SJ, Yong MC, et al. Improved efficacy of neoadjuvant compared to adjuvant immunotherapy to eradicate metastatic disease. Cancer Discov 2016;6:1382–99. https://doi.org/10.1158/2159-8290.CD-16-0577.

203. Siegler EL, Wang P. Preclinical models in chimeric antigen receptor-engineered T-cell therapy. Hum Gene Ther 2018;29:534–46. https://doi.org/10.1089/hum.2017.243.

204. Puchalapalli M, Zeng X, Mu L, et al. NSG mice provide a better spontaneous model of breast cancer metastasis than Athymic (Nude) Mice. PLoS One 2016;11:e0163521. https://doi.org/10.1371/journal.pone.0163521.

205. Walsh NC, Kenney LL, Jangalwe S, et al. Humanized mouse models of clinical disease. Annu Rev Pathol 2017;12:187–215. https://doi.org/10.1146/annurev-pathol-052016-100332.

206. Wang M, Yao LC, Cheng M, et al. Humanized mice in studying efficacy and mechanisms of PD-1-targeted cancer immunotherapy. FASEB J 2018;32:1537–49. https://doi.org/10.1096/fj.201700740R.

207. Brehm MA, Cuthbert A, Yang C, et al. Parameters for establishing humanized mouse models to study human immunity: analysis of human hematopoietic stem cell engraftment in three immunodeficient strains of mice bearing the IL2rgamma(null) mutation. Clin Immunol 2010;135:84–98. https://doi.org/10.1016/j.clim.2009.12.008.

208. DeRose YS, Wang G, Lin YC, et al. Tumor grafts derived from women with breast cancer authentically reflect tumor pathology, growth, metastasis and disease outcomes. Nat Med 2011;17:1514–20. https://doi.org/10.1038/nm.2454.

209. Gonzalez L, Strbo N, Podack ER. Humanized mice: novel model for studying mechanisms of human immune-based therapies. Immunol Res 2013;57:326–34. https://doi.org/10.1007/s12026-013-8471-2.

210. King MA, Covassin L, Brehm MA, et al. Human peripheral blood leucocyte non-obese diabetic-severe combined immunodeficiency interleukin-2 receptor gamma chain gene mouse model of xenogeneic graft-versus-host-like disease and the role of host major histocompatibility complex. Clin Exp Immunol 2009;157:104–18. https://doi.org/10.1111/j.1365-2249.2009.03933.x.

Biotech and Breakthroughs in Immuno-Oncology

Jeffrey M. Bockman, PhD

KEYWORDS

- Immunotherapy • Immuno-oncology • Checkpoint inhibitors • Tumor microenvironment
- Urologic oncology

KEY POINTS

- Paradigm-shift in disease management with the approval of immuno-oncology agents, namely, checkpoint inhibitors, created a major shift in how patients with cancers are treated.
- The significant clinical impact of checkpoint inhibitors led to what some have seen as a goldrush, others as a bubble, toward clinical development of immunotherapies.
- Immuno-oncology agents have not by and large cured most patients in most cancers, hence new immunotherapeutic agents and combinations are needed.
- Over the past 5 years, much of the BioPharma industry's focus has been on expanding the range of immuno-oncology agents and combinations.

The age of immunotherapy has been a century in the making, from the first published reports of Dr Coley through the approvals in the late 1980s, of interferon-alpha in hairy cell leukemia, follicular non-Hodgkin lymphoma, melanoma, and AIDS-related Kaposi sarcoma, to the approvals in the early 1990s of IL-2 for and metastatic renal cell carcinoma (RCC) and melanoma, to the long-standing standard of care use of Bacillus of Calmette and Guerin in non–muscle-invasive bladder cancer and formal approval by the US Food and Drug Administration in 1990 for carcinoma in situ of the bladder. Over this time, despite these approvals and notwithstanding the problematic therapeutic index of these agents and generally limited efficacy, the belief in the role of the immune system fighting off cancer remained by and large suspect within the pharmaceutical industry. Those scientists and clinicians researching and believing in the potential, known then as "tumor immunologists," worked against the prevailing dogma of direct killing of cancer cells, whether by radiation, chemotherapy, or later "targeted" therapies, ranging from early antibodies like *Herceptin* (trastuzumab) for HER2$^+$ breast cancer and rituximab

(Rituxan) for CD20$^+$ non-Hodgkin's lymphoma or small molecule mostly kinase inhibitors like imatinib (Gleevec) targeting bcr-abl fusions for chronic myeloid leukemia and erlotinib (Tarceva) for epidermal growth factor receptor-driven non–small cell lung cancer (NSCLC).

With the approvals of sipuleucel-T (Provenge), the first cancer vaccine approved in the United States, for prostate cancer, and ipilimumab, anti-CTLA-4 (Yervoy), the first checkpoint inhibitor (CPI) approved in the world, both in 2011, followed by the first anti-programmed death 1 (PD-1) CPIs approved in 2014, nivolumab (Opdivo) and pembrolizumab (Keytruda), so begins the new age of immunotherapy as not only a validated anticancer approach but as a significant blockbuster category within the pharmaceutical industry (**Fig. 1**).

As shown in **Fig. 1**, sales of leading oncology drugs worldwide, one can readily see the extent to which the anti–PD-1 and anti–PD-ligand 1 agents define the immuno-oncology (IO) space now and going forward over the next 5 years, and in fact by 2024 pembrolizumab becomes the largest pharmaceutical product in the world, surpassing the anti-inflammatory anti-tumor necrosis

Oncology Practice Head, Cello Health Bio Consulting (Previously Defined Health), 25-B Hanover Road, Suite 320, Florham Park, NJ 07932, USA
E-mail address: jbockman@cellohealth.com

Urol Clin N Am 47 (2020) 511–521
https://doi.org/10.1016/j.ucl.2020.07.006

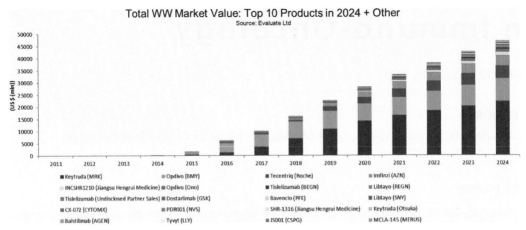

Fig. 1. Sales of leading immuno-oncology agents. (*From* EvaluatePharma, Cello Health BioConsulting (previously Defined Health) analysis.)

factor product adalimumab (Humira) that has been the biggest selling drug for some time. Nivolumab becomes the fourth-leading product.

That pembrolizumab and nivolumab are among the top selling pharmaceutical products is significant because it reflects the degree to which this class of immunotherapy agents, the CPIs, have become a new foundational component of therapeutic regimens across multiple tumor types.

Such a role for CPIs is akin to that of the taxanes like paclitaxel (Taxol) and docetaxel (Taxotere) in the first decades of the modern age of oncology. CPIs are approved or in development for a wide range of tumors. Most activity is in solid tumors, especially those with good clinical activity and extent approvals, such as melanoma, NSCLC, and the urologic oncology indications of RCC and bladder cancer (**Fig. 2**).

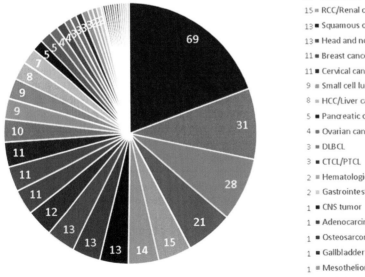

Fig. 2. CPIs in clinical development across all cancers. CTCL, cytotoxic T-cell lymphoma; DLBCL, diffuse large B-cell lymphoma; HCC, hepatocellular carcinoma; PTCL, peripheral T-cell lymphoma; RCC, renal cell carcinoma. (*From* Adis R&D Insight, Clarivate Analytics Cortellis, Cello Health BioConsulting (previously Defined Health) analysis.)

Number of Assets in Clinical Development	Cancer	Solid Tumor	GBM/Glioma	Neuroblastoma	CNS Tumor	Head and Neck Cancer	Breast Cancer	Ovarian Cancer	Cervical Cancer	Endometrial Cancer	Prostate Cancer	Penis Tumor	RCC/Renal Cancer	Bladder Cancer	Colorectal Cancer	NSCLC	Small Cell Lung Cancer	Mesothelioma	Melanoma	Merkel Cell Carcinoma	Squamous Cell Carcinoma	Pancreatic Cancer	Gallbladder Cancer	Biliary Cancer	HCC/Liver Cancer	Esophageal Cancer	Gastric Cancer	Gastrointestinal Cancer	Osteosarcoma	Soft Tissue Sarcoma	Adenocarcinoma	Cancer Metastases
PD-1	2	19				4	1	2	4		1		5	8	4	9	4		9	2	4				4	3	3	1		1		1
PD-L1	1	18				1	2		3	1	1	1	2	6	3	8	1		3	1	2	2	1	3	1	1		1				
LAG-3	1	4	1			2		1	1	1			1	1		2	1	1	1	1					1	1	1				1	
PD-L1 / 4-1BB		4				2			1	1			1	2		2			1		1				1	1	1					
TIGIT		5					1	1					1	1	1	2			1		1				1		1					
PD-1 / CTLA-4	1	3				1	1		1				1	1	1	2			1	1	1				1	1	1				1	
CTLA-4 / LAG-3		1				2	1		1	1			1	1	1	1	1		1		1	1			1	1	1					
PD-1 / ICOS		1				1	1		1	1			1	1	1	1			1		1	1	1		1	1	1					
CTLA-4		4												1		1	2	1	5													
TIM-3	3	5																														
PD-L1 / CTLA-4	1	1				1								1					1						1							
PD-1 / DLL1													1		1	1			1		1											
B7-H3		2		1	1																											
PD-1 / TIM-3		1														1		1														
PD-1 / PD-L1		2														1																
NKG2A						1										1																
VISTA	1																															
CTLA-4 / OX40		1																														
PD-L1 / TGF-B		1																														
PD-L1 / VISTA	1																															
LAG-3 / PD-L1																																
KIR			1																													1
TIM-3 / PD-L1		1																														
CTLA-4 / CD80		1																														
PD-1 / OX-40L		1																														
PD-1 / LAG-3	1																															
Undefined	1																															

Legend
Highest Count Key
1   5   10   15   20

Fig. 3. Heat map of immunomodulatory antibodies across cancer settings. HCC, hepatocellular carcinoma; RCC, renal cell carcinoma. (*From* Adis R&D Insight, Clarivate Analytics Cortellis, Cello Health BioConsulting (previously Defined Health) analysis.)

As shown in **Fig. 3**, a heat map of the count of currently marketed and development stage immunomodulatory antibodies, one can readily see the intense competitive clinical development in the validated setting of anti–PD-1/ligand 1 inhibitors, as well as the high level of activity in next-generation CPIs against new targets and that of the costimulatory agonists of various classes. The excitement around immunotherapies, or IO as the space is increasingly referred to, is reflected in various analytics of pipeline and clinical trial activity. As our analysis shows (**Fig. 4**), the clinical development pipeline is increasingly a diverse range of IO targets and therapeutic modalities.

The intensity of IO development, specifically around the anti–PD-1/PD-ligand 1 agents, is underscored in the analysis by the Cancer Research Institute of clinical trials from 2017 to 2019. As shown in **Fig. 5**, combinations studies of the now 9 approved CPIs is nearly 3000 active studies. Such competitive intensity starts with patient enrollment and continues into the clinical development strategy and ultimately commercialization, with extensive investment by the leading CPI players in life cycle management to expand

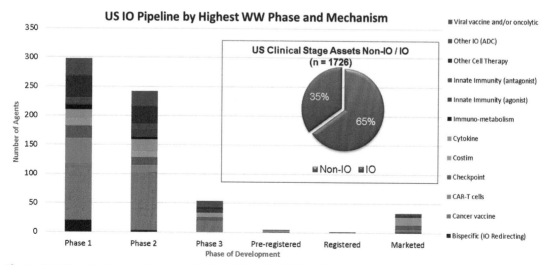

Fig. 4. Oncology clinical development pipeline (US only). ADC, antibody-drug conjugate. (*From* Adis R&D Insight, Clarivate Analytics Cortellis, Cello Health BioConsulting (previously Defined Health) analysis.)

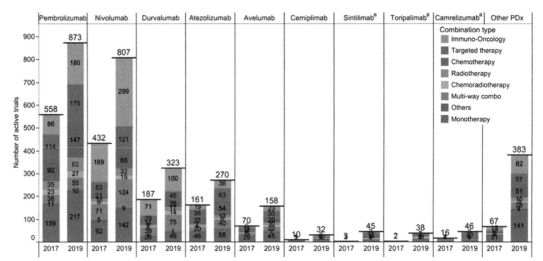

Fig. 5. Clinical trials with CPIs, 2017 versus 2019. [a] Approved in China only. PDx, products. (*From* Jia Xin Yu, Jeffrey P. Hodge, Cristina Oliva, Svetoslav T. Neftelinov, Vanessa M. Hubbard-Lucey & Jun Tang. Trends in clinical development for PD-1/PD-L1 inhibitors. Nature Reviews Drug Discovery 19, 163-164 (2020); with permission.)

the labels by settings within indications (vertical franchise expansion) and across more tumor types (horizontal franchise expansion).

The sheer number of combination trials highlights both the strengths and weaknesses of the CPIs: they have been paradigm-changing in selected settings for 20% to 60% of patients, in tumors like melanoma and NSCLC, but they are not working in all patients even in the more "immunoresponsive" or "hot" cancers and there are key, high unmet need cancers like pancreatic, where they have little to no activity, the so-called "cold" tumors. Hence, the need for layering on other agents with overlapping and distinct mechanisms of action (MOA), both IO agents and, if we may use the colloquial coinage, "non-IO" agents. As

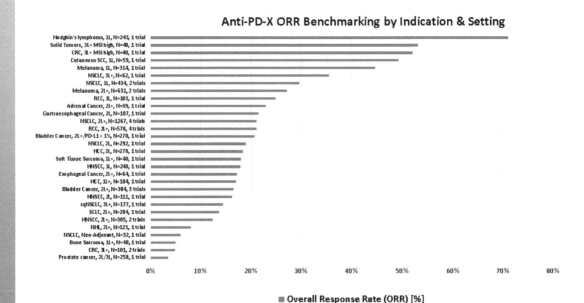

Fig. 6. Aggregate overall response rates (ORR) per tumor type and line of therapy across monotherapies. CRC, colorectal cancer; HCC, hepatocellular carcinoma; HNSCC, head and neck squamous cell carcinoma; MSI, microsatellite instability; SCC, squamous cell carcinoma; SCLC, small cell lung cancer. (*From* Adis R&D Insight, Clarivate Analytics Cortellis, Beacon Targeted Therapies, Cello Health BioConsulting (previously Defined Health) analysis.)

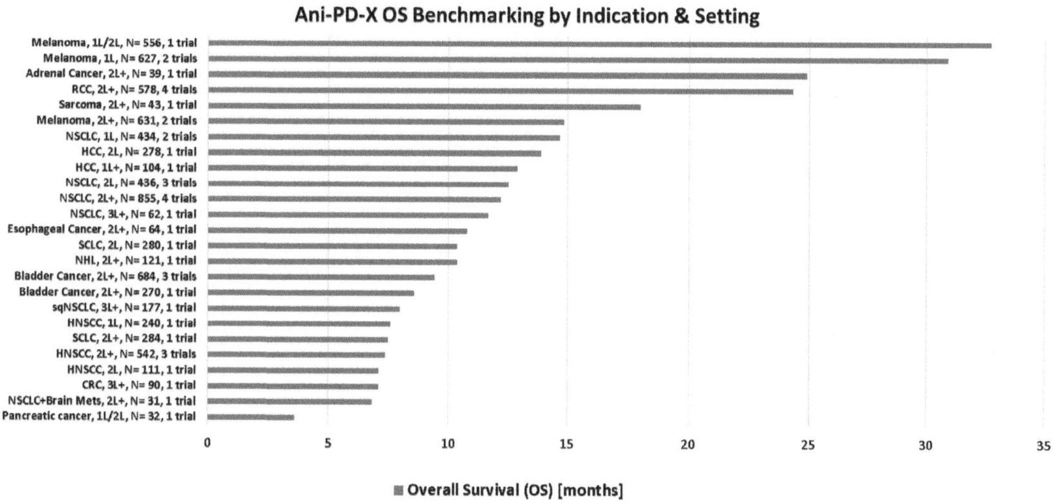

Ani-PD-X OS Benchmarking by Indication & Setting

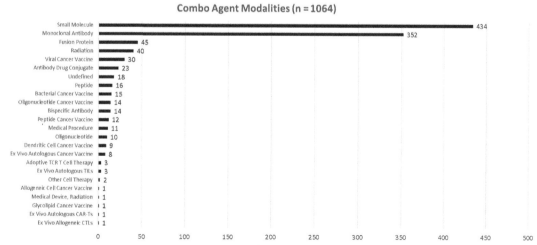

Overall Survival (OS) [months]

Fig. 7. Aggregate overall survival (OS) per tumor type and line of therapy across monotherapies. CRC, colorectal cancer; HCC, hepatocellular carcinoma; HNSCC, head and neck squamous cell carcinoma; NHL, non-Hodgkin lymphoma; SCLC, small cell lung cancer. (*From* Adis R&D Insight, Clarivate Analytics Cortellis, Beacon Targeted Therapies, Cello Health BioConsulting (previously Defined Health) analysis.)

Figs. 6 and **7** show in terms of the clinical activity of CPIs, the range of efficacy as expressed by overall response rate or my overall survival with CPIs varies widely, from low single digit to nearing 70% overall response rate for monotherapy use, and from more than 30 months in melanoma to less than 5 months for pancreatic cancer as a monotherapy.

As is readily apparent, RCC is near the top of the more immunoresponsive cancers, bladder, at least for activity of CPIs, is in the lower middle (but is muddied by specific setting of bladder cancer and line, such as whether it is Bacillus of Calmette and Guerin refractory), and at the other end of the spectrum is prostate cancer, one of the least immunoresponsive tumors. It is worth noting, however, that prostate cancer was the first tumor type to get an IO agent approved since the times of IL-2 and interferon, and although melanoma is as expected near the top, the activity of CPIs in NSCLC was really not anticipated, although in retrospect through the lens of tumor mutational burden, this now makes sense.

As one can see in **Fig. 8**, cold tumors are being heavily studied in combination with CPIs, especially small molecule combinations.

Combo Agent Modalities (n = 1064)

Fig. 8. Combinations by therapeutic modality. CAR-Ts, chimeric antigen receptor technology; CTLs, cytotoxic T cells; TCR, T-cell receptor. (*From* Adis R&D Insight, Clarivate Analytics Cortellis, Beacon Targeted Therapies, Cello Health BioConsulting (previously Defined Health) analysis.)

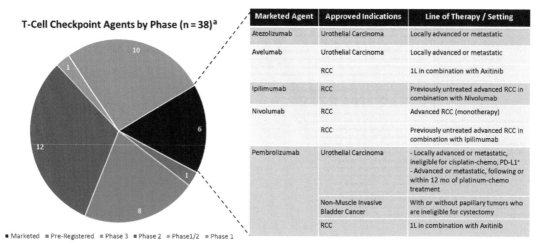

T-Cell Checkpoint Agents by Phase (n = 38)[a]

Marketed Agent	Approved Indications	Line of Therapy / Setting
Atezolizumab	Urothelial Carcinoma	Locally advanced or metastatic
Avelumab	Urothelial Carcinoma	Locally advanced or metastatic
	RCC	1L in combination with Axitinib
Ipilimumab	RCC	Previously untreated advanced RCC in combination with Nivolumab
Nivolumab	RCC	Advanced RCC (monotherapy)
	RCC	Previously untreated advanced RCC in combination with Ipilimumab
Pembrolizumab	Urothelial Carcinoma	- Locally advanced or metastatic, ineligible for cisplatin-chemo, PD-L1⁺ - Advanced or metastatic, following or within 12 mo of platinum-chemo treatment
	Non-Muscle Invasive Bladder Cancer	With or without papillary tumors who are ineligible for cystectomy
	RCC	1L in combination with Axitinib

■ Marketed ■ Pre-Registered ■ Phase 3 ■ Phase 2 ■ Phase1/2 ■ Phase 1

Fig. 9. Leading CPIs, from Phase 1 through Marketed for top 3 urology settings of kidney, prostate and bladder cancers. [a] Products in development for multiple indications are double-counted. (*From* Adis R&D Insight, Clarivate Analytics Cortellis, Cello Health BioConsulting (previously Defined Health) analysis.)

Turning now specifically to analysis of the oncology and IO for urologic cancers, as **Fig. 9** shows, this has been an active area for CPI approvals, with 5 unique programs currently approved and several others in late-stage development. Of course, the activity includes life cycle management among the 5 agents shown that are approved in urologic cancers, as well as the marketed CPIs not yet approved in any urologic setting, and follow-on CPIs not yet approved for any indication.

Looking at all clinical development activity in oncology for the 3 lead indications of kidney, bladder, and prostate cancers (**Fig. 10**), the snapshot of the pipeline reflects substantive activity for

immunotherapy agents versus "nonimmunotherapy" programs. In fact, there is more IO activity as a percentage in these 3 indications than broadly for oncology overall (43% vs 35%, respectively; see **Fig. 4**). The diversity of overall anticancer approaches is not unexpected, with cell signaling kinase inhibitors, epigenetic inhibitors, hormonal modulation, antiangiogenics, and still a good and quite active development of cytotoxic agents (next generation, reformulations, drug delivery, etc).

Diving more specifically into the pipeline for each of these 3 main tumor types, as shown in **Fig. 11**, one can see a large bolus of phase II agents IO agents that are moving toward

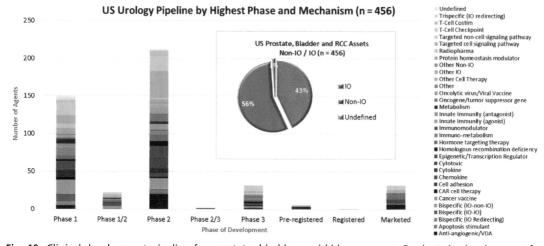

Fig. 10. Clinical development pipeline for prostate, bladder, and kidney cancers. Products in development for multiple indications are double counted. VDA, vascular disrupting agent. (*From* Adis R&D Insight, Clarivate Analytics Cortellis, Cello Health BioConsulting (previously Defined Health) analysis.)

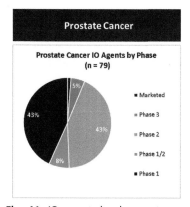
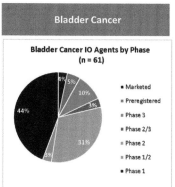
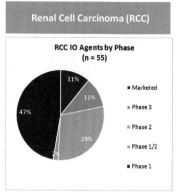

Fig. 11. IO agent development across the prostate, bladder and kidney cancer indications. (*From* Adis R&D Insight, Clarivate Analytics Cortellis, Cello Health BioConsulting (previously Defined Health) analysis.)

registration. As shown in the next several figures of our analytics, many of the IO agents for urologic cancers, as is true of the broad IO pipeline, whether CPIs or other MOAs, are looking to combine with small molecule kinase inhibitors of various sorts and with multiple chemotherapy agents regimens.

Antibodies are the leading therapeutic modality for development across the leading urologic cancers (**Fig. 12**). And although small molecule agents are generally the second most common approach, cancer vaccines remain a major focus of development; in fact, in prostate cancer it is the most active IO modality. That cancer vaccines remain such an active category in prostate cancer may reflect their safety profile and the ability to position them at either end of the spectrum from earlier stage disease, for example, as a maintenance adjunctive to an androgen receptor antagonist, or in late stage disease where the therapeutic

options are more limited and patient's performance status more compromised.

As an example of these combination approaches, **Fig. 13** shows late stage agents for RCC. As is evident, IO agent, primarily anti–PD-1 or anti–PD-ligand 1, are being combined with validated MOAs like antiangiogenic agents, which may also have immunomodulatory effects on the tumor microenvironment, as well as novel targets like inhibitors of c-met, given hepatocyte growth factor (HGF)/mesenchymal epithelial transition factor (c-MET) seems to have a an immunosuppressive role in through the direct inhibition of dendritic cells and an indirect inhibition of T-cell proliferation.

Fig. 14 shows a comparable analysis for prostate cancer, but of the entire clinical stage pipeline. There is a fairly robust pipeline with a few promising agents on the immediate horizon. Of note, there is increasing trial focus on targeted therapies

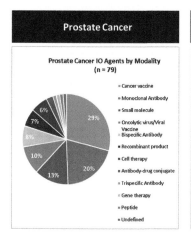
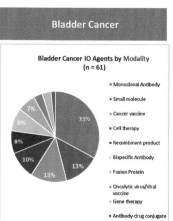
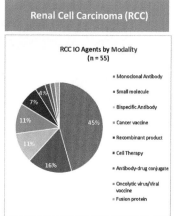

Fig. 12. IO pipeline activity in prostate, bladder, and kidney cancer indications. (*From* Adis R&D Insight, Clarivate Analytics Cortellis, Cello Health BioConsulting (previously Defined Health) analysis.)

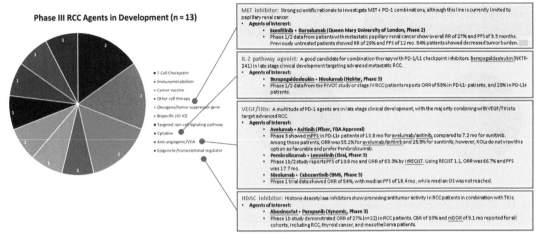

Fig. 13. Late stage RCC programs. FDA, US Food and Drug Administration; HDAC, histone deacetylase; KLOs, key opinion leaders; mDORs, mouse delta-opioid receptors; RR, relative risk; TKI, tyrosine kinase inhibitor; VDA, vascular disrupting agent; VEGF, vascular endothelial growth factor. (*From* Adis R&D Insight, Clarivate Analytics Cortellis, Cello Health BioConsulting (previously Defined Health) analysis and Primary Research. https://ir.nektar.com/news-releases/news-release-details/preliminary-data-nktr-214-combination-opdivo-nivolumab-patients, https://ascopubs.org/doi/abs/10.1200/JCO.2019.37.15_suppl.3022, https://ascopubs.org/doi/abs/10.1200/JCO.2019.37.7_suppl.545?af=R, https://ascopubs.org/doi/abs/10.1200/JCO.2018.36.15_suppl.4560, https://ascopubs.org/doi/abs/10.1200/JCO.2018.36.6_suppl.515, www.ClinicalTrials.gov, Cancer Discov. 2019; 9(6):711:721. J. Clin. Onco. 2018; 36(15). NEJM 2019; 380:1103-1115.)

and IO/non-IO combinations, as well as biomarker-selected, late stage programs for metastatic castrate-resistant prostate cancer including 177Lu-PSMA-617 for PSMA + patients, ipatasertib for PTEN-negative patients, and PARP inhibitors for homologous repair–deficient patients.

Last, I turn to some of the deals and investments that have been going into IO, because this reflects

opportunities for academics and their institutions to put into a proper context potential early stage collaborations or new company ("newco") formation. In viewing IO through the twin lenses of investing and deal-making perspective, some interesting trends become apparent (**Fig. 15**).

First and foremost, what strikes one looking at these metrics is the size of the investments in IO

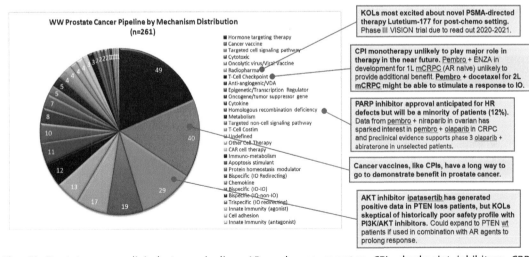

Fig. 14. Prostate cancer clinical stage pipeline. AR, androgen receptor; CPI, checkpoint inhibitors; CRPC, castration-resistant prostate cancer; KLOs, key opinion leaders; mCRPC, metastatic castration-resistant prostate cancer; PSMA, prostate-specific membrane antigen; VDA, vascular disrupting agent. (*From* Adis R&D Insight, Clarivate Analytics Cortellis, Cello Health BioConsulting (previously Defined Health) analysis and Primary Research.)

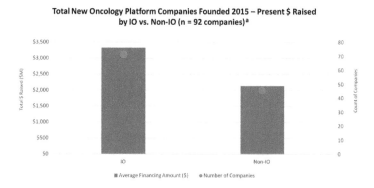

Fig. 15. Oncology company investments (indication agnostic). [a] Companies with platform(s) that are applicable to both IO or non IO approaches are double counted. Only venture funding data points were used to calculate the total amount raised. (*From* BCIQ, Cello Health BioConsulting (previously Defined Health) analysis.)

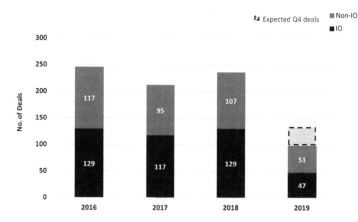

Fig. 16. IO deal making 2016 to quarter 3 of 2019. (*From* BCIQ, Cello Health BioConsulting (previously Defined Health) analysis.)

Top 10 Deals by Upfront Value ($M): 2018						
Rank	Company	Deal Partner/ Product Source	Product(s)	Phase	Upfront[a]	Milestones	Total (Upfront + Milestones)
1	Celgene	Juno Therapeutics	Multiple	Phase 1/2	9,000	Undisclosed	9,000
2	GSK	Tesaro	Multiple	Marketed	5,100	Undisclosed	5,100
3	Sanofi	Ablynx N.V	Multiple	Registration	4,800	Undisclosed	4,800
4	Servier	Shire	Pegaspargase, Multiple	Marketed	2,400	Undisclosed	2,400
5	Novartis	Endocyte	Multiple	Registration	2,100	Undisclosed	2,100
6	Bristol-Myers Squibb	Nektar Therapeutics	NKTR-214	Phase 3	1,850	1,800	3,650
7	Eli Lilly	Armo Biosciences	Multiple	Phase 3	1,600	Undisclosed	1,600
8	Seattle Genetics	Cascadian Therapeutics	Multiple	Phase 3	614	Undisclosed	614
9	Johnson & Johnson	Argenx S.E	Cusatuzumab	Phase 2	500	1,300	1,800
10	Merck & Co.	Viralytics	Cavatak	Phase 2	371	Undisclosed	371

Top 10 Deals by Total Value ($M): 2018						
Rank	Company	Deal Partner/ Product Source	Product(s)	Phase	Upfront[a]	Milestones	Total (Upfront + Milestones)
1	Celgene	Juno Therapeutics	Multiple	Phase 1/2	9,000	Undisclosed	9,000
2	Merck & Co.	Eisai	Lenvatinib mesylate	Marketed	300	4,385	5,785
3	GSK	Tesaro	Multiple	Marketed	5,100	Undisclosed	5,100
4	Genentech	Affimed N.V.	Multiple	NA	96	4,950	5,046
5	Sanofi	Ablynx N.V	Multiple	Registration	4,800	Undisclosed	4,800
6	Bristol-Myers Squibb	Nektar Therapeutics	NKTR-214	Phase 3	1,850	1,800	3,650
7	Gilead	Sangamo	Multiple	Preclinical	150	3,000	3,150
8	Allogene Therapeutics	Pfizer	UCART19	Phase 1	0	185	2,800
9	Shire	Servier	Pegaspargase, Multiple	Marketed	2,400	0	2,400
10	Novartis	Endocyte	Multiple	Registration	2,100	Undisclosed	2,100

Contains IO program

Fig. 17. Top deals in 2018 as grouped by IO and non IO. [a] Upfront includes upfront cash and upfront equity; NA (not applicable) = can include deals with multiple agents or portfolio where phase is not applicable. (*From* BCIQ, Evaluate Pharma, Cello Health BioConsulting (previously Defined Health) analysis.)

Top 10 Deals by Upfront Value ($M): 2019							
Rank	Company	Deal Partner/ Product Source	Product(s)	Phase	Upfront[a]	Milestones	Total (Upfront + Milestones)
1	BMS	Celgene	Multiple	NA	35,000	Undisclosed	74,000
2	Pfizer	Array BioPharma	Multiple	NA	11,400	Undisclosed	11,400
3	Eli Lilly	Loxo Oncology	Multiple	NA	7,234	Undisclosed	7,234
4	AstraZeneca	Daiichi Sankyo	Trastuzumab deruxtecan	Phase 3	1,350	5,550	6,900
5	Merck & Co.	Peloton Therapeutics	Multiple	NA	1,050	1,150	2,200
6	GSK	Merck KGaA	Bintrafusp alfa (M7824)	Phase 2	344	3,871	4,214
7	Merck & Co.	Immune Design	Multiple	NA	248	Undisclosed	248
8	Clinigen Group	Novartis AG	Proleukin, aldesleukin (Macrolin)	Marketed	180	30	210
9	Amgen	Nuevolution AB	Multiple	NA	167	Undisclosed	167
10	Aurobindo Pharma	Spectrum Pharmaceuticals	Multiple	NA	160	140	300

Top 10 Deals by Total Value ($M): 2019							
Rank	Company	Deal Partner/ Product Source	Product(s)	Phase	Upfront[a]	Milestones	Total (Upfront + Milestones)
1	BMS	Celgene	Multiple	NA	35,000	Undisclosed	74,000
2	Pfizer	Array BioPharma	Multiple	NA	11,400	Undisclosed	11,400
3	Eli Lilly	Loxo Oncology	Multiple	NA	7,234	Undisclosed	7,234
4	AstraZeneca	Daiichi Sankyo	Trastuzumab deruxtecan	Phase 3	1,350	5,550	6,900
5	GSK	Merck KGaA	Bintrafusp alfa (M7824)	Phase 2	344	3,871	4,214
6	Abpro Corporation	Chia Tai Tianqing Pharmaceutical	Multiple	NA	Undisclosed	Undisclosed	4,000
7	Gilead	Nurix Therapeutics	Multiple	NA	45	2,300	2,345
8	Merck	Peloton Therapeutics	Multiple	NA	1,050	1,150	2,200
9	Codiak BioSciences	Jazz Pharmaceuticals	Multiple	NA	56	Undisclosed	1,076
10	Cytovant Sciences	Medigene AG	Multiple	NA	10	1,000	1,010

Contains IO program

Fig. 18. Top deals in 2019 as grouped by IO and non IO. [a] Upfront includes upfront cash and upfront equity; NA (not applicable) = can include deals with multiple agents or portfolio where phase is not applicable. (*From* BCIQ, Evaluate Pharma, Cello Health BioConsulting (previously Defined Health) analysis.)

over the past 5 years, with roughly 50% more money raised and more companies funded for IO-centric platform companies than non-IO ones. Although these analyses are not specific to urologic cancers, but rather to oncology broadly, nevertheless the general conclusion seems to be that the appeal of immunotherapy within the health care ecosystem remains strong.

As shown in **Fig. 16**, IO deals actually slowed in 2019, with less than 50% of the prior year, raising the question of whether a spate of failures (IDO inhibitors, for example) has led to some maturing in understanding and a higher bar, or just fatigue in IO along with a renewed interest, perhaps owing to this fatigue, in non-IO options.

However, a drill down into the data reveals a somewhat more nuanced picture. Using the top deals, licensing or M&A, as a surrogate of industry interest, the years 2015 to 2018 displayed intense "IO frenzy" with the majority of the top deals as

defined by total deal value (which includes upfront and milestones, plus any equity) or simply by the size of the upfront payments would be categorized as IO. Looking only at 2018, for example, in **Fig. 17**, it is clear the extent to which deals in the IO space commanded more real and prospective dollar value than non-IO deals.

However, using this same approach to look at 2019 (**Fig. 18**), one might conclude that perhaps some maturing of vision has begun, with a more balanced view of the need for diverse IO and non-IO approaches to tackle cancer. The apparent renewed interest in non-IO options reflects in part a return to precision medicine agents (eg, NTRK inhibitors from LOXO, for example). Many in the industry have observed that the intense focus in IO spurred by the clinical (and financial) performance of the CPIs ultimately led to a situation within the BioPharma and investor community where these successes overshadowed some important

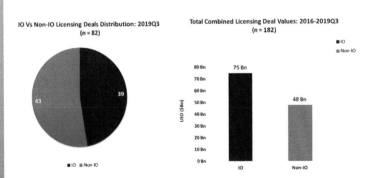

Fig. 19. Total licensing deals and value, 2016 to quarter 3 of 2019, by IO and non IO. *Note left graph = all counts include undisclosed and missing deal values, whereas the right graph excludes them. (*From* BCIQ, Cello Health BioConsulting (previously Defined Health) analysis.)

2018 Venture (Seed & Series A) Financing
Distribution
$2.23B Total Raised in 2018

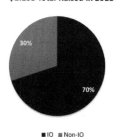

■ IO ■ Non-IO

2019 To-Date Venture (Seed & Series A)
Financing Distribution
$0.73B Total Raised in 2019

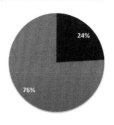

■ IO ■ Non-IO

Fig. 20. Venture funding in oncology, seed and series A, 2016 to quarter 3 of 2019, by IO and non IO. (*From* BCIQ, Cello Health BioConsulting (previously Defined Health) analysis.)

limitations of the rush into the space, such that business strategy overruled translational science, leading to a number of clinical trial stumbles we have seen with novel MOAs attempting to follow in the footsteps of the CPIs.

Looking cumulatively from 2016 through the third quarter of 2019, one can see how the number of IO and non-IO deals were nearly equal, but the total deal value for IO was more than 50% greater than for non-IO deals (**Fig. 19**). This underscores the hope, and the hype, around immunotherapies being true paradigm changing therapies. However, as noted elsewhere in this article, there was a noticeable change from 2018 to 2019 in oncology funding and startups (series A and seed), essentially an inversion from being IO dominant in 2018 to being non-IO dominant in 2019, while at the same time far less monies were invested into oncology in 2019. Although certainly macro trends drove the overall lower investment in oncology newcos, the switchover from IO to non IO again highlights a potential realignment, what might be called a return to a more reasoned and balanced (in terms of MOAs) investing strategy (**Fig. 20**).

In conclusion, for all the successes that the CPIs have had over the past 9 years since their first approvals, and all the industry noise around partnerships and newcos in IO, it can seem at times that more of the talk is around what is not working in IO. The high-profile failure of the IDO inhibitors, along with underperformance or safety issues with other novel MOAs being combined with CPIs, has added a strain of skepticism to what some had long felt to be an overhyped space. Thinking of this rather as the maturing of the field, the issue remains as to how best to move novel IO programs forward. Certainty, a reemphasis on reasonable single-agent activity is a the top of correctives, but there is still more to be done in more fully interrogating the biology and doing the translational work around these novel targets and pathways, their role in combination with CPIs, and how best to position them for clinical development and for optimal patient benefit.

DISCLOSURE

CHBC works for many BioPharma companies developing immuno-oncology therapies on a project fee basis. Neither I nor the company has any financial stake in any of these clients.

Special Article

Personalized Medicine for the Infertile Male

Danielle Velez, MD[a], Kathleen Hwang, MD[b],*

KEYWORDS

- Male infertility • Personalized medicine • Proteomics • Genomics

KEY POINTS

- Personalized medicine uses a patient's genotype, environment, and lifestyle choices to create a tailored diagnosis and therapy plan, with the goal of minimizing side effects, avoiding lost time with ineffective treatments, and guiding preventative strategies.
- Sir William Osler, one of the founding fathers of Johns Hopkins Hospital, recognized that "variability is the law of life, and as no two faces are the same, no two bodies are alike, and no two individuals react alike, and behave alike under the abnormal conditions we know as disease."[1]
- The study of the -omics: proteomics, genomics, lipomics, and so forth, is yielding an array of new biomarkers to characterize the type of infertility and detect and/or monitor genetic changes, possibly from environmental factors.

INTRODUCTION

Sir William Osler, one of the founding fathers of Johns Hopkins Hospital, recognized that "variability is the law of life, and as no two faces are the same, no two bodies are alike, and no two individuals react alike, and behave alike under the abnormal conditions we know as disease."[1] Centuries later, Sir Osler's hope for personalized medicine is ready to take the center stage in health care. Personalized medicine uses a patient's genotype to tailor further diagnostic testing and therapies to minimize side effects, avoid lost time with ineffective treatments, and guide preventative strategies. The mapping of the human genome in 2003, the discovery of single nucleotide polymorphisms (SNPs) and advances in RNA microarrays have facilitated advancement in the study of the "-omics:"

- Genomics: study of genes and their function
- Proteomics: study of proteins
- Metabolomics: study of molecules involved in cellular metabolism

- Transcriptomics: study of mRNA
- Glycomics: study of cellular carbohydrates
- Lipomics: study of cellular lipids
- Spermatogenesomics: comprehensive study of all factors affecting spermatogenesis

Fig. 1 illustrates the transition from a "one-size-fits-all" approach to that of precision medicine.[2] By considering each patient's unique characteristics, ranging from genetics to lifestyle choices, the goal of personalized medicine is to choose and administer therapy plans in a more rapid and targeted fashion, minimizing the margin for error or failure. Personalized medicine has already made its way from the laboratory bench to the patient's bedside. Four percent to 5% of patients with cystic fibrosis have the G551D mutation in the cystic fibrosis transmembrane conductance regulator gene (CFTR), causing the CFTR-driven ion gate to remain closed, resulting in excess pulmonary mucus production.[3] Ivacaftor is a Food and Drug Administration–approved medication for children as young as 6 months of age with the G551D mutation. In patients with colorectal

[a] Division of Urology, Department of Surgery, Brown University, 2 Dudley Street Suite 185, Providence, RI, USA;
[b] Department of Urology, University of Pittsburgh School of Medicine, Pittsburgh, PA, USA
* Corresponding author. Division of Urology, University of Pittsburgh Medical Center, 3471 Fifth Avenue, Suite 700, Pittsburgh, PA.
E-mail address: hwangky@upmc.edu

Urol Clin N Am 47 (2020) 523–536
https://doi.org/10.1016/j.ucl.2020.07.003

Current Medicine
One Treatment Fits All

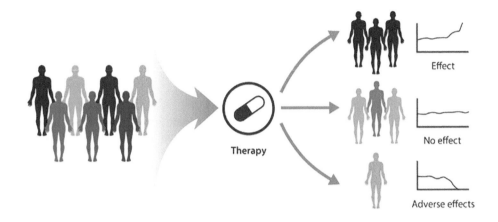

Future Medicine
More Personalized Diagnostics

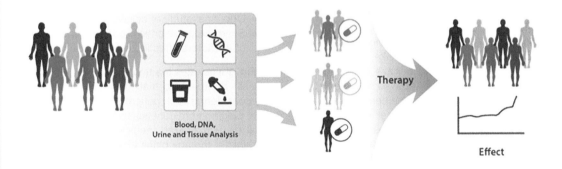

Fig. 1. Comparison of the current model for medicine versus the future personalized model. (*From* Barbeau J. PDX and Personalized Medicine. Crown Bioscience blog. 2018. Available at: https://blog.crownbio.com/pdx-personalized-medicine. Accessed March 13, 2020; with permission.)

cancer, somatic mutations in the PIK3CA gene are associated with improved cancer-specific survival with postoperative aspirin.[2]

Within reproductive endocrinology, preimplantation genetic diagnosis and screening (PGD, PGS, respectively) are widely offered to couples to diagnose or to screen for undesired genetic diseases. The PGD International Society estimates greater than 100,000 cycles have been performed over the last 23 years. Most PGD is for aneuploidy testing, to improve in vitro fertilization (IVF) outcomes in patients with recurrent pregnancy loss, or for those who have failed IVF.[4] In cases of a

family history of X-linked diseases, PGD has been used to select for female embryos, to avoid genetic disease in male offspring. In 2004, it was estimated ~1000 children had been born after undergoing PGD/PGS, to at-risk parents, with the same prevalence of congenital malformations as the general population.[5]

Personalized medicine is being promoted and embraced by physicians, politicians, and patients. In 2007, then President Barak Obama created the Genomic and Personalized Medicine Act, providing funding for the advancement of precision medicine. The United States Department of

Health and Human Services also issued a Personalized Health Care directive to increase the usefulness and application of genomic knowledge. With government financial support and new research being published and presented by physicians and scientists every year, patients can expect to benefit from targeted diagnostics, preventative strategies, and more effective therapies.

STANDARD MALE INFERTILITY WORKUP: WHAT IS THE STANDARD MALE INFERTILITY WORKUP

Infertility is defined as an inability to achieve pregnancy after at least 12 months of regular, unprotected intercourse. It occurs in ~15% of couples, with male infertility accounting for the primary or combined cause in 50%.[6] The evaluation of the infertile man includes a thorough history and physical examination to identify abnormalities in the testes, vas deferens, or seminal vesicles, as well as risk factors for infertility, such as a history of cryptorchidism, testicular trauma or infections, or a family history of infertility. Testing begins with 2 semen analyses, performed after 1 to 3 days of abstinence and at least 2 to 3 weeks apart. The World Health Organization[7] has established standard ranges of normal, based on population studies:

- Sperm concentration: ≥15 million sperm per milliliter of semen
- Sperm volume: greater than 39 million
- Semen volume: ≥1.5 mL
- Morphology: greater than 4% normal form
- Motility: ≥40%

Specific abnormalities in the semen analysis, when present in both samples, will prompt varying workups. Moderate oligospermia (concentration ≤10 million/mL) prompts an endocrine evaluation, with a total testosterone, follicle-stimulating hormone (FSH), and luteinizing hormone, whereas severe oligospermia (concentration ≤5 million/mL) requires a karyotype and evaluation for Y-chromosome microdeletion assay. For men without any sperm, or azoospermia, the above tests help to distinguish between obstructive and nonobstructive azoospermia (NOA).

However, the semen analysis is not a perfect test. Couples with normal semen analyses are still unable to spontaneously conceive, and conversely, men with abnormal semen analyses may have normal fertility. Ultimately, the most common diagnosis in male infertility is idiopathic.[8]

When an infertility-related disease is identified, there are few therapies to directly treat the cause of the infertility. Rather, couples rely on assisted reproductive technologies to bypass the cause in favor of the desired result: intrauterine insemination or IVF, with or without intracytoplasmic injection (ICSI). For men without sperm in the ejaculate, sperm is acquired via epididymal or testicular extraction, which may be performed either in the office with local anesthesia or in the operating room under a general anesthetic. However, if sperm cannot be identified, such as in Sertoli cell–only (SCO) syndrome patients, whereby successful sperm extraction is at best 44.5%, as reported by a tertiary-care, high-volume center,[9] couples are left with the options of donor sperm or adoption.

At its core, fertility is the successful combination of the genetic material of a solitary egg and sperm, and then uterine implantation of the embryo. Every step in this process is guided by genetics, and as evidenced by the treatment approach discussed above, male infertility is not well suited for a "one-size-fits-all" approach. Ultimately, this makes the study of male infertility a unique niche for the application of personalized medicine.

SPERMATOGENESIS FAILURE: THE FUTURE FOR SPERMATOGONIA STEM CELL TRANSPLANTATION AND GENOMIC EDITING

Spermatogenesis failure may be endocrine (testosterone production) or exocrine (sperm production) derived. Medical management for endocrine spermatogenesis failure is well established, including supplemental luteinizing hormone, recombinant human FSH, selective estrogen receptor modulators, and aromatase inhibitors.[10] Traditionally, there have been few management options for dysfunctional spermatogonial stem cells (SSC), which are required for self-renewal and differentiation into mature sperm. Examples of this include patients who are status-post chemotherapy and/or radiation, those with maturation arrest, or SCO syndrome, which includes Klinefelter syndrome and AZF microdeletions.[11] Without functional SSCs, patients present with NOA and are dependent on surgical sperm extraction with eventual IVF/ICSI to achieve fatherhood. In addition, patients may require PGD to prevent NOA inheritance in offspring.

Although the above is a solution, it does not correct the root of the problem. Successful spermatogenesis requires spermatogonia proliferation, spermatocyte development, and spermatid differentiation. Failure at any point in this process results in impaired infertility.[12] In a review of testicular biopsy samples in 534 men undergoing infertility evaluation, only 3.2% showed normal histology and spermatogenesis. Maturation arrest was present in 34% of the patients, hypospermatogenesis in 32%, and SCO syndrome in 16%.[13] Repopulating the testis with functional cells through spermatogonial stem cell transplantation (SSCT), with the added possibility of germline genomic editing to correct for disease-causing mutations, is a burgeoning area of research for spermatogenesis failure.[14]

SSCT has thus far yielded healthy offspring in rodents. Wu and colleagues[15] demonstrated that SSCs, cryopreserved for 12 to 14 years, could be implanted into adult male mice testes, previously treated with alkylating agent busulfan. Two months after transplantation, the number and length of spermatogenesis colonies were equivalent between freshly isolated and cryopreserved cells. Sperm heads were isolated from the recipient testes of cryopreserved SSCs, and ultimately yielded 5 healthy pups, of whom two were produced by natural mating. Furthermore, these pups were fertile and produced fertile generations that appeared normal.

There are several challenges with translating this research to humans. In pediatric oncology patients requiring gonadotoxic chemoradiation therapy, there may be more than 14 years between tissue harvesting and desire for fertility, in which time possible genetic and epigenetic abnormalities may be incurred. Furthermore, there are a limited number of SSCs derived from the small testis biopsies, requiring in vitro expansion before transplantation. Thus far, human SSCs have shown successful propagation in mouse testes, but have yet to be demonstrated in large animal models.[13] SSCT depends on the identification and isolation of normal SSCs, which must survive the freezing and thawing process. Finally, SSCT of flawed SSC may still result in impaired spermatogenesis (ie, maturation arrest), or inheritance of genetic defects that may render future offspring infertile (ie, Y-chromosome microdeletions). However, several advances have been made in the identification of specific genes contributing to male infertility, as well as genomic editing.

Genomic abnormalities affect approximately 15% of infertile patients with azoospermia or severe oligospermia. Currently, these men are recommended a very limited genetic workup, namely a karyotype and testing for Y-chromosome microdeletions, in addition to an endocrine evaluation.[16] This workflow has largely remained the same for more than 15 years, and unfortunately, up to 70% of men will be diagnosed with idiopathic male-factor infertility. Genome-wide association studies have focused on identifying genes that cause or contribute to spermatogenic failure. These candidate genes can then be considered targets for genomic editing. Cannarella[17] created a complete list of 60 genes thought to cause human spermatogenesis failure (Table 1). The authors expect the number of target genes to continue to grow. With further multicenter studies, the hope is that these genes will be linked to findings on the semen analysis (ie, asthenospermia, vs globoozospermia, or cryptospermia), which will then narrow the number of genes tested.

If the first step to treating male infertility is to identify the cause, then the next step is to repair the defect. Engineered, site-specific nucleases carry the possibility of genetically modified SSCs, which would overcome fertility obstacles, as well as prevent the passage of inheritable diseases to future generations. Zinc-finger nucleases (ZFNs), transcription-activator-like effector nucleases (TALENs), or the RNA-guided clustered regularly interspaced short palindromic repeat (CRISPR-Cas9 system) generated DNA double-stranded breaks at specific sites. The break may be repaired by error-prone nonhomologous end joining, or by more precise homology-directed repair (HDR), which depends on a repair template of DNA that complements the flanking area of injury, to control what is inserted into the break.[18]

ZFNs were the first platform for genomic editing. Using chimeric proteins and an endonuclease, the zinc finger can bind to ~3 nucleotides, which activates the endonuclease to create a break in the DNA. The break is then repaired as explained above. The ZFN is time-intensive to engineer, and although both halves of the ZFN must recognize the DNA sequence, there is known off-target activity, which has the possibility of disastrous outcomes down the line if used in SSCs.

TALENs use effector proteins from the Xanthomonas bacterial species. The DNA binding domain consists of ~34 amino acids, with a key number 12 to 13 amino acid, named the repeat variable dinucleotide (RVD). The RVD is highly variable and changes to it dictate which DNA sequence is bound. In this way, the TALEN is more highly versatile and easily engineered than the ZFN. However, it is still subject to off-target activity and is not as reliable or efficacious as the CRISPR-Cas9 nuclease system.

CRISPR-Cas9 is derived from Streptococcus pyogenes and relies on a single-guide RNA (sgRNA) for site-specific DNA recognition and cleavage, and an endonuclease (Cas9). The sequence-specific targeting element (crRNA), which is integrated into the sgRNA, recognizes and pairs with a DNA length of ~20 to 60 nucleotides. The targeting of this area of DNA depends on a protospacer adjacent motif (PAM), which is present in nearly every gene, at multiple sites,

Table 1
Genes involved in human spermatogenic failure

Gene Name	Full Name	MIM Number	Infertility Phenotype	Cytogenetic Location	References
AK7	*Adenylate kinase 7*	615364	Flagella abnormalities	14q32.2	Lores et al, 2018
AURKC	*Aurora kinase C*	603495	Macrozoospermia	19q 13.43	Ben Khelifa et al, 2011
BRDT	*Bromodomain, testis-specific*	602144	Acephalic spermatozoa	1p22.1	Li et al, 2017
CATSPER1	*Cation channel, sperm-associated, 1*	606389	Oligozoospermia	11q13.1	Avenarius et al, 2009
CCDC39	*Coiled-coil domain-containing protein 39*	613798	Oligoasthenozoospermia. Flagella abnormalities	3q26.33	Ji et al, 2017
CEP135	*Centrosomal protein, 135 kDa*	611423	Flagella abnormalities	4q12	Sha et al, 2017a, b, Tang et al, 2017, Coutton et al, 2018
CFAP43	*Cilia- and flagella-associated protein 43*	617558	Flagella abnormalities	10q25.1	Sha et al, 2017a, b, Tang et al, 2017, Coutton et al, 2018
0CFAP44	*Cilia- and flagella-associated protein 44*	617559	Flagella abnormalities	3q13.2	Sha et al, 2017a, b
CFAP69	*Cilia- and flagella-associated protein 69*	617949	Flagella abnormalities	7q21.13	Dong et al, 2018
DAZ1	*Deleted in azoospermia 1*	400003	NOA	Yq11.223	Foresta et al, 1999, Mozdarani et al, 2018
DAZ2	*Deleted in azoospermia 2*	400026	NOA	Yq11.223	Foresta et al, 1999, Mozdarani et al, 2018
DAZ3	*Deleted in azoospermia 3*	400027	NOA	Yq11.23	Foresta et al, 1999, Mozdarani et al, 2018
DAZ4	*Deleted in azoospermia 4*		NOA	Yq11.223	Foresta et al, 1999, Mozdarani et al, 2018
DBY (DDX3Y)	*DeadlH Box 3, Y-linked*	400010	NOA (spermatocytes maturation arrest)	Yq11.221	Foresta et al, 2000
DMCl	*Disrupted meiotic Cdna 1, yeast, homolog of*	602721	NOA	22q13.1	He et al, 2018
DMRTl	*Doublesex- andMAB3-related transcription factor 1*	602424	NOA	9p24.3	Lopes et al, 2013, Tewes et al, 2014. Tuttelmann et al, 2018

(continued on next page)

Table 1
(continued)

Gene Name	Full Name	MIM Number	Infertility Phenotype	Cytogenetic Location	References
DNAAFI	*Dynein, axonemal, assembly factor 1*	613190	Flagella abnormalities	16q24.1	Ji et al, 2017
DNAAF2	*Dynein, axonemal, assembly factor 2*	612517	Asthenozoospermia. Flagella abnormalities	14q21.3	Ji et al, 2017
DNAAF3	*Dynein, axonemal, assembly factor 3*	614566	Flagella abnormalities	19q13.42	Ji et al, 2017
DNAHI	*Dynein, axonemal, heavy chain 1*	603332	Flagella abnormalities	3p21.1	Ben Khelifa et al, 2014, Amiri-Yekta et al, 2016, Wang et al, 2017, Tang et al, 2017
DNAH5	*Dynein, axonemal, heavy chain 5*	603335	Asthenozoospermia, flagella abnormalities	5p15.2	Ji et al, 2017
DNAH6	*Dynein, axonemal, heavy chain 6*	603336	NOA (spermatocytes maturation arrest) Globozoospermia, acephalic spermatozoa	2p11.2	Gershoni et al, 2017, Li et al, 2018a, b
DNAI1	*Dynein, axonemal, intermediate chain 1*	604366	Asthenozoospermia. flagella abnormalities	9p13-p21	Ji et al, 2017
DNAI2	*Dynein, axonemal, intermediate chain 2*	605483	Flagella abnormalities	17q25	Ji et al, 2017
DNAJB13	*DNAJ/HSP40 homolog, subfamily B, member 13*	610263	Flagella abnormalities	11q13.4	El Khouri et al, 2016
DPY19L2	*DPY19-like 2*	613893	Globozoospermia	12q14.2	Koscinski et al, 2011, Harbuz et al, 2011, Ellnati et al, 2012
DYXIC1 (DNAAF4)	*Dynein axonemal assembly factor 4*	608706	Asthenozoospermia, flagella abnormalities	15q21.3	Ji et al, 2017
FANCM	*FANCM gene*	609644	NOA	14q21.2	Kasak et al, 2018, Yin et al, 2018
FS1P2	*Fibrous sheath-interacting protein 2*	615796	Flagella abnormalities	2q32.1	Martinez et al, 2018
HAUS7	*Haus Augmin-like complex, subunit 7*	300540	Oligozoospermia	Xq28	Li et al, 2018a, b

Gene	Gene name	OMIM	Phenotype	Location	Reference
HEATR2 (DNAAF5)	Heat repeat-containing protein 2	614864	Flagella abnormalities	7p22.3	Ji et al, 2017
HSF2	Heat shock-transcription factor 2	140581	NOA (spermatocytes maturation arrest)	6q22.31	Mou et al, 2013
HYD1N	Hydrocephalus-inducing, mouse, homolog of	610812	Asthenozoospermia	16q22.2	Ji et al, 2017
KLHL10	Kelch-like 10	608778	Oligozoospermia	17q21.2	Yatsenko et al, 2006
LRRC6	Leucine-rich repeat-containing protein 6	614930	Asthenozoospermia, flagella abnormalities	8q24.22	Ji et al, 2017
ME10B	Meiosis-specific protein with OB domains	617670	NOA (spermatocytes maturation arrest)	16p13.3	Gershoni et al, 2017
NR5A1	Nuclear receptor subfamily 5, group A, member 1	184757	NOA (spermatocytes maturation arrest), oligozoospermia	9q33.3	Bashamboo et al, 2010, Ferlin et al, 2015
P1H1D3	PIH1 domain-containing protein 3	300933	Flagella abnormalities	Xq22.3	Paff et al, 2017
PLK-4	Polo-like kinase 4	605031	NOA	4q28.l	Miyamoto et al, 2016
RSPH1	Radial spoke head 1, Chlamydomonas, homolog of	609314	Flagella abnormalities	21q22.3	Ji et al, 2017
RSPH4A	Radial spoke head 4A, Chlamydomonas, homolog of	612647	Flagella abnormalities	6q22.1	Ji et al, 2017
RSPH9	Radial spoke head 9, Chlamydomonas, homolog of	612648	Flagella abnormalities	6p21.2	Ji et al, 2017
SEPT 12	Septin 12	611562	OAT	16p13.3	Kuo et al, 2012
SLC26A8	Solute carrier family 26 (sulfate transporter), member 8	608480	Asthenozoospermia	6p21.31	Dirami et al, 2013
SOHLH1	Spermatogenesis- and oogenesis-specific basic helix-loop-helix protein 1	610224	NOA	9q34.3	Choi et al, 2010, Nakamura et al, 2017
SPATA 16	Spermatogenesis-associated protein 16	609856	Globozoospermia	3q26.31	Dam et al, 2007
SPINK2	Serine protease inhibitor, Kazal-type, 2	605753	NOA, OAT	4q12	Kherraf et al, 2017
SUNS	SAD1 and UNC84 domain-containing protein 5	613942	Acephalic spermatozoa	20q11.21	Zhu et al, 2016

(continued on next page)

Table 1
(continued)

Gene Name	Full Name	MIM Number	Infertility Phenotype	Cytogenetic Location	References
SYCE1	*Synaptonemal complex central element protein 1*	611486	NOA	10q26.3	Maor-Sagie et al, 2015, Huang et al, 2015
SYCP3	*Synaptonemal complex protein 3*	604754	NOA	12q23.2	Stouffs et al, 2005a, b
TAF4B	*TAF4B RNA polymerase II, TATA Box-binding protein-associated factor*	601689	NOA, oligozoospermia	18q11.2	Ayhan et al, 2014
TDRD6	*Tudor domain-containing protein 6*	611200	OAT	6p12.3	Sha et al, 2018a, b, c
TEX 11	*Testis-expressed gene 11*	300311	NOA (spermatocytes maturation arrest)	Xq13.1	Yatsenko et al, 2015, Sha et al, 2018a, b, c
TEX14	*Testis-expressed gene 14*	605792	NOA	17q22	Gershoni et al, 2017
TEX15	*Testis-expressed gene 15*	605795	NOA	8q12	Okutman et al, 2015, Colombo et al, 2017
TSGA10	*Testis-specific protein 10*	607166	Acephalic spermatozoa	2q11.2	Sha et al, 2018a, b, c
USP26	*Ubiquitin-specific protease 26*	300309	NOA	Xq26.2	Ma et al, 2016
WDR66	*WD repeat-containing protein 66*	618146	Flagella abnormalities	12q24.31	Kherraf et al, 2018
ZMYND10	*Zinc finger mind-containing protein 10*	607070	Flagella abnormalities	3q21.31	Ji et al, 2017
ZMYND15	*Zinc finger mind-containing protein 15*	614312	NOA (spermatocytes maturation arrest)	17p13.2	Ayhan et al, 2014

Abbreviation: OAT, oligoasthenoteratozoospermia.

From Cannarella, R et al. New insights into the genetics of spermatogenic failure: a review of the literature. *Human Genetics* 2019(138):125–140; with permission.

giving the CRISPR-Cas9 nuclease its advantage over TALEN or ZFNs.

Fig. 2 shows the construction of sgRNA and donor DNA, and **Fig. 3** illustrates HDR-mediated gene editing.[19] sgRNA are designed to create double-stranded breaks (DSB) within the target DNA (see **Fig. 2**B), and then single-stranded DNA (ssDNA) oligo insertions are introduced: point (see **Fig. 2**C), short fusion tag (see **Fig. 2**D), or a larger fragment of circular DNA (see **Fig. 2**E). These ssDNA oligos are flanked by 40- to 60-bp sequences on either side, with the required PAM (in this case, 5′-NGG). The 40- to 60-bp sequences are homologous to the sequence surrounding the sgRNA-mediated DSB, thus guiding the ssDNA oligo to the break site for insertion.

In comparison to ZFNs and TALEN, the CRISPR system has been tested on modified SSCs with genome-wide screens, without obvious off-target genetic changes. The system has enabled rapid genomic editing in various species, including correcting the CFTR locus in cultured intestinal stem cells of cystic fibrosis patients.[20] Wu and colleagues[21] demonstrated the ability to apply the CRISPR-Cas9 system to modify the CRYGC gene in SSCs, which were then transplanted into the seminiferous tubules of infertile mice. Subsequent round spermatids were injected into

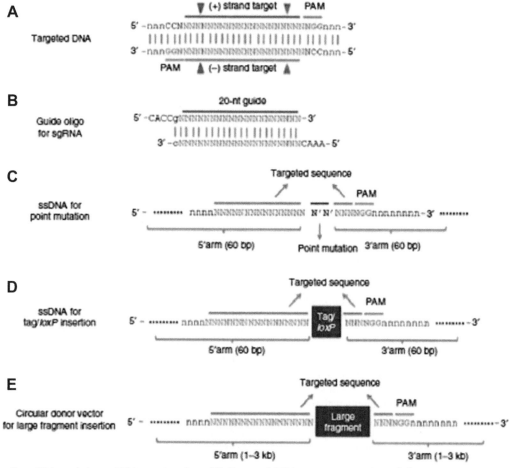

Fig. 2. sgRNA and donor DNA construction. (*A*) Targeted DNA sequence consists of the DNA target (*red bar*) directly upstream of a requisite 5′-NGG adjacent motif (PAM; *green*). Cas9 mediates a DSB ~3 bp upstream of the PAM for the (+) strand (*blue triangle*) or (−) strand (*red triangle*). (*B*) The guide oligos contain overhangs for ligation, a G-C base pair (*blue*) added at the 5′ end of the guide sequence for T7 transcription and the 20-bp sequence preceding the 5′-NGG in genomic DNA. (*C*) ssDNA for point mutation consists of a point-mutation site (*purple*), flanked by 60-bp sequences on each side adjoining the DSBs. (*D*) ssDNA for tag/*loxP* insertion consists of the purple site, flanked by 60-bp sequences on each side adjoining the DSBs. (*E*) A circular donor vector for large fragment insertion consists of a large fragment, flanked by homology arm sequences on each side adjoining the DSBs. (*From* Yang, H et al. Generating genetically modified mice using CRISPR/Cas-mediated genome engineering. *Nature Protocols.* 2014; with permission.)

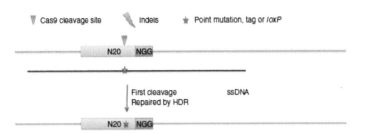

Fig. 3. HDR-mediated gene editing by an *ssDNA* template at a DSB created by Cas9. (*From* Yang, H et al. Generating genetically modified mice using CRISPR/Cas-mediated genome engineering. *Nature Protocols.* 2014; with permission.)

oocytes, and 100% of the resultant offspring were born with the corrected phenotype. The CRISPR-Cas9 has the advantage of greater efficiency in targeting genomic loci, because several sgRNAs may be used to increase the number of targeted genes.[18]

As referenced earlier in this article, repopulating the testes with a higher density of SSCs is not enough to achieve fertility if the maturation into normal spermatids is not possible. The *c-kit* gene is highly conserved and plays a vital role in male germ cell development. Any mutation in the gene is likely to result in maturation arrest, because of the inability of the SSC to complete meiosis.[22] Yuan and colleagues[22] used TALEN to modify a point mutation in *c-kit*, with resultant normal spermatogenesis from the modified SSCs, which were transplanted back into mouse testes.

Combining the above, men with SSCs, isolated from either prepubertal testis biopsies or during their adult workup for male-factor infertility, have the potential for normal parenthood, through SSC transplantation, with or without correction of genetic mishaps via germline genomic editing. Although the research to support these efforts is still within the laboratory, intensive efforts are underway to progress the science to reality.

SEMINAL PLASMA (PROTEOMICS)

Personalized medicine is not just the search for a therapeutic plan unique to the individual patient. It is also aimed at grouping patients within a spectrum of disease to allow for more targeted diagnostic testing and therapies, with the goal of minimizing the likelihood of ineffective or even harmful treatment. The study of the -omics, or the characterization and quantification of biological molecules, which are central to precision medicine research, is uniquely applied to the field of male infertility, whereby the intricacies of cellular biology, genetics, proteins, and cell signaling are center stage.

Seminal plasma is an easily acquired medium, but one that is rarely studied within male infertility. It is known to contain high levels of lipids, proteins,

sugars, and metabolites that intimately interact with the spermatozoa, supporting the acrosome reaction, fertilization, and oocyte interaction.[23] It holds great promise as a possible source of infertility biomarkers, particularly in men with underlying azoospermia. Currently, azoospermia is diagnosed by routine semen analysis, used in the context of a thorough history, physical examination, and endocrine evaluation. To date, however, there are no noninvasive tests to predict the likelihood of zero spermatogenic reserve within the testes.[24] Patients must instead endure a negative testicular exploration. Thus, there has been great interest in identifying a noninvasive biomarker for the diagnosis of NOA secondary to spermatogenic failure.

Seminal plasma contains high concentrations of small extracellular vesicles (sEVs), which contain noncoding RNA, such as microRNA (miRNAs). The miRNAs in particular appear to vary according to the sEVs' cell of origin; therefore, the type of miRNA present within the sEV reflects the pathophysiology of the origin organ.[25] Furthermore, because miRNA are bound to protein complexes and/or contained within the sEV, they cannot cross the blood-testis barrier, making the seminal plasma miRNA a possible biomarker for the pathophysiology of testicular cells.[23] Barceló and colleagues[24] analyzed exosome miRNA levels in seminal plasma from normozoospermic, fertile men, postvasectomy men, men with NOA, and men with severe oligospermia. Of 623 miRNAs that were studied, 1 miRNA (miR-31-5p) was found to have greater than 90% sensitivity and specificity in distinguishing between obstructive azoospermia and NOA, with a greater area under the curve than even plasma FSH (0.957, $P<.0001$ vs 0.85, $P = .004$). With further validation, seminal plasma miRNA is a future tool for urologists to identify men with a real possibility of sperm extraction and recovery for IVF/ICSI.

Protein expression in seminal plasma has also been studied in relation to the level of oxidative stress and reactive oxygen species (ROS). Although elevated ROS has been implicated as a cause of male infertility, data correlating levels of

ROS to pregnancy and live birth outcomes are limited.[15] However, the seminal plasma is rich in molecules that support spermatozoa function; therefore, a greater understanding of the relationship between these proteins and ROS may provide new avenues for male infertility diagnosis and treatment. Using proteomic assays, Sharma and colleagues[26] found proteins unique to men with elevated levels of ROS that were involved in cell morphology, motility, aging, and differentiation, suggesting that these proteins may play a role in apoptosis and necrosis. Wang and colleagues[27] studied the presence of metalloids within the seminal plasma, noting that rising quartiles of seminal arsenic and cadmium were associated with poor sperm motility, whereas a positive correlation was found between seminal zinc and sperm concentration. These studies are examples of novel research using seminal plasma properties, rather than sperm characteristics, to view male infertility, with the ultimate goal being improved diagnostics and more effective therapies.

EPIGENETICS (EPIGENOMICS)

The human genome is made up of DNA, which is a blueprint for proteins to carry out cell functions. The epigenome is a variety of chemical compounds that direct the genome to produce specific proteins. DNA methylation is an epigenetic mechanism, whereby an additional methyl body (CH_3) is added to DNA, ultimately changing that specific gene expression by inhibiting transcription. Expression of noncoding RNAs is another epigenetic mechanism known to contribute to male fertility.[28] Changes to the epigenome are much more dynamic, undergoing changes over years and generations, rather than the human genome, which is relatively stable. Therefore, identification of epigenome-based markers has become an important complement to traditional genetic markers. DNA methylation vastly differs between tissues, but often the disease-specific target tissues are difficult to access or minimally available, such as in the testis. Peripheral blood-based DNA markers have been studied as a close proxy and have already proven useful for cancer diagnosis and prognosis, diabetes, and other diseases.[29]

Two studies have examined peripheral blood-based DNA markers for male infertility. Friemel and colleagues[28] analyzed DNA methylation signatures in 30 infertile and 10 fertile men, using HumanMethylation450 BeadChip. They identified 471 CpG loci that were methylated only in the infertile group, of which 26 did not match to a known SNP. These 26 loci correlated to 15 genes,

of which 4 could be linked to male fertility. ENO1 codes for alpha enolase, which has been identified as a marker for sperm fertility in animal studies. MTA2 encodes proteins exclusively expressed by Sertoli cells, and LBX2 and BRSK2 are both expressed in testicular tissue, although their exact role in spermatogenesis remains unclear. The authors chose to focus on 2 other genes, PIWIL1 and PIWIL2, because the piwi-interacting RNA binding proteins are known to have a major role in spermatogenesis. PIWIL 1 controls translation late in spermatogenesis, and PIWIL is required for germline stem cell line renewal. They found the infertile group had substantially higher average DNA methylation rates compared with fertile controls for PIWIL 1 and PIWIL 2: 60% versus 26%, and 80% versus 40%, respectively. With higher rates of methylation, these genes are not expressed; knockout of these genes in mouse models results in infertile mice. Other studies have noted PIWIL2 methylation is associated with lower sperm count[30] and spermatogenic failure.[31]

Sarkar and colleagues[29] supported the above with their own analysis of peripheral blood DNA methylation values in fertile versus infertile men. The investigators identified 170 genes that significantly differed in methylation patterns between the 2 groups, of which 38 played a role in spermatogenesis, including PDHA2, which has a role in sperm energy metabolism, and FHIT, which is involved in testicular germ cell maturation and differentiation. Cross-referencing the Friemel data, there were 52 differentially methylated CpGs (DMCs) in common between the German and Indian study populations. These 52 DMCs represent potential methylation-based markers for male infertility. Ultimately, more studies are needed to validate these findings in other populations.

SUSCEPTIBILITY GENES TO ENVIRONMENTAL FACTORS IN MALE INFERTILITY

There is a burgeoning field of research into the impact of environmental factors on the epigenome. Variations in diet, lifestyle, chemical exposure, and even medications have been linked to major pathologic conditions, such as cancer, obesity, diabetes, and cardiovascular disease. The effect of environmental exposure and lifestyle on reproductive health is still poorly understood but certainly represents an opportunity for personalized medicine in the treatment of male infertility. As previously described, genetic expression is heavily influenced by epigenetic changes, namely histone modifications and methylation patterns. These epigenetic markers are reset at multiple points from male germ cell development, to the creation of an embryo, and even through puberty.[32] Susceptibility genes are those which are altered by the environment, which may result in disease in the patient or even subsequent offspring.

Men who smoke have been reported to have higher levels of sperm DNA damage,[33] which may result in infertility or recurrent pregnancy loss. Maternal nutrition has been extensively studied and has resulted in creation of prenatal vitamins and other guidelines to minimize risk of infectious disease and neurologic congenital malformations in children. Fewer, if any, guidelines exist for paternal diet. Furthermore, nutrition is known to be tied to epigenetic changes. In studying the agouti viable yellow mouse model, Waterland and Jirtle[34] found that methyl donor supplementation for the gestating mother can directly change the degree of methylation upstream of the agouti gene, thereby changing the pup hair color from salt/pepper to yellow.

Gametic differentially methylated regions are areas within the genome that are not expressed, because of hypermethylation of 1 parental allele. Epigenetic markers, including histone modifications and methylation patterns, are reset at multiple points in the male reproductive cycle, from male germ cell development, to the creation of an embryo, and even through puberty. These changes are susceptible to environmental factors, with higher rates of rare genetic imprinting disease, such as Beckwith-Wiedemann syndrome, or Angelman syndrome, occurring in IVF/ICSI children. Epigenetic changes have been linked to cell culture medium, embryo freezing, timing of embryo transfer, and maternal exposure to high doses of gonadotropins.[35]

In addition to IVF/ICSI, there are many other environmental/lifestyle factors that are thought to impact the reproductive epigenome. Persistent organic pollutants (POPs) were widely used until the 1980s, but are so chemically stable that food supplies continue to be exposed. Many POPs have been found to have a toxic effect on the reproductive and endocrine systems, including sperm quality, spermatic DNA integrity, and hormone levels.[34] Fetal exposures to dibutyl and diethylhexyl phthalates had cumulative and dose-dependent effects of anatomic malformations within the reproductive tract, such as epididymal agenesis and delayed Leydig cell differentiation, cryptorchidism, and hypospadias.

As more of these pathologic gametic differentially methylated regions are identified, the obvious next research area must be treatment focused. Given the vulnerability of male and female reproductive health to environmental factors, nutrition, hormone exposures, and other lifestyle represent opportunities to repair reproductive pathologic condition not only for the patient but also for subsequent generations.

SUMMARY

Both personalized medicine and fertility are anchored in the human genome, and although some parts of precision medicine have much maturing to do within the research laboratory, other aspects have found a place in the infertility clinic, offering options to couples seeking to build their family. The infertility workup has remained largely unchanged and poorly diagnostic. Treatment that gets to the root of the infertility issue is also lacking, with reliance on IVF/ICSI as a workaround to achieving pregnancy. In spermatogenesis failure, SSC therapy may become an opportunity for men with even the smallest amounts of sperm extracted, or with a history of sperm banking, to repopulate the testis, such that their partner may avoid hormonal manipulation in IVF/ICSI. PGD/PGS is well established within infertility clinics, but as CRISPR is further developed, embryos may be pretreated rather than selected, thereby minimizing the risk of IVF/ICSI and embryo harm, and preventing inheritance of the genetic disorder in subsequent generations. Genome-wide association studies are searching for genes contributing to spermatogenic failure. Eventually these genes should be linked to findings on the semen analysis, so the semen analysis can be used as a stepping stone to more directed genetic testing, and eventually therapy, possibly with genomic editing. The study of the -omics: proteomics, genomics, lipomics, and so forth, is yielding an array of new biomarkers to characterize the type of infertility and detect and/or monitor genetic changes, possibly from environmental factors. Seminal plasma and peripheral blood are the new targets of these studies, being the easiest to acquire. Biomarkers within miRNA, DNA methylation levels and locations, and histone changes have been identified, but the data must be validated in different populations. Many research questions remain: will these new biomarker tests be cost-effective? What is the ideal population for these tests? After the tests are validated and widely available, will treatments be available for the diagnoses? What are the ethics involved in genetic testing and editing?

Much like other areas like oncology or immunology, by focusing on the genome, precision medicine is an opportunity to ask more specific questions and tailor therapies in a streamlined fashion to minimize side effects and ineffective treatments, while producing durable results for patients. With government and industry support, the old protocolized methodology is soon to be replaced.

REFERENCES

1. Ginsburg GS, Willard HF. Genomic and personalized medicine: foundations and applications. Transl Res 2009;154(6):277–87.
2. Barbeau J. PDX and personalized medicine. In: Crown Bioscience blog. 2018. Available at: https://blog.crownbio.com/pdx-personalized-medicine. Accessed March 13, 2020.
3. Goetz LH, Schork NJ. Personalized medicine: motivation, challenges, and progress. Fertil Steril 2018; 109(6):952–63.
4. Stern H. Preimplantation genetic diagnosis: prenatal testing for embryos finally achieving its potential. J Clin Med 2014;3(1):280–309.
5. Verlinsky Y, Cohen J, Munne S, et al. Over a decade of experience with preimplantation genetic diagnosis: a multicenter report. Fertil Steril 2004;82(2): 292–4.
6. Thoma ME, McLain AC, Louis JF, et al. Prevalence of infertility in the United States as estimated by the current duration approach and a traditional constructed approach. Fertil Steril 2013;99(5):1324–31. e1.
7. Cooper TG, Noonan E, Eckardstein SV, et al. World Health Organization reference values for human semen characteristics*‡. Hum Reprod Update 2010;16(3):231–45.
8. Sigman M. Evaluation of the sub-fertile male. St Louis (MO): Mosby; 1997.
9. Berookhim BM, Palermo GD, Zaninovic N, et al. Microdissection testicular sperm extraction in men with Sertoli cell–only testicular histology. Fertil Steril 2014;102(5):1282–6.
10. Ramasamy R, Stahl PJ, Schlegel PN, et al. Medical therapy for spermatogenic failure. Asian J Androl 2012;14(1):57–60.
11. Cunha M. Y-chromosome microdeletions in nonobstructive azoospermia and severe oligozoospermia. Asian J Androl 2017;19(3):338.
12. Hentrich A, Wolter M, Szardening-Kirchner C, et al. Reduced numbers of Sertoli, germ, and spermatogonial stem cells in impaired spermatogenesis. Mod Pathol 2011;24(10):1380–9.
13. McLachlan RI, Rajpert-De Meyts E, Hoei-Hansen CE, et al. Histological evaluation of the human testis–approaches to optimizing the clinical value of the assessment: mini review. Hum Reprod 2006;22(1):2–16.
14. Mulder CL, Zheng Y, Jan sZ, et al. Spermatogonial stem cell autotransplantation and germline genomic editing: a future cure for spermatogenic failure and prevention of transmission of genomic diseases. Hum Reprod Update 2016;22(5):561–73.
15. Wu X, Goodyear SM, Abramowitz LK, et al. Fertile offspring derived from mouse spermatogonial stem cells cryopreserved for more than 14 years. Hum Reprod 2012;27(5):1249–59.
16. Jarow J. The optimal evaluation of the infertile male: AUA best practice statement. 2010.
17. Cannarella R. New insights into the genetics of spermatogenic failure: a review of the literature. Hum Genet 2019;138(2):125–40.
18. Costa JR, Bejcek BE, McGee JE, et al. Genome Editing Using Engineered Nucleases and Their Use in Genomic Screening. 2017 Nov 20. In: Sittampalam GS, Grossman A, Brimacombe K, et al, editors. Assay Guidance Manual [Internet]. Bethesda (MD): Eli Lilly & Company and the National Center for Advancing Translational Sciences; 2004. Available at: https://www.ncbi.nlm.nih.gov/books/NBK464635/.
19. Yang H, Wang H, Jaenisch R, et al. Generating genetically modified mice using CRISPR/Cas-mediated genome engineering. Nat Protoc 2014; 9(8):1956–68.
20. Schwank G, Koo BK, Sasselli V, et al. Functional Repair of CFTR by CRISPR/Cas9 in intestinal stem cell organoids of cystic fibrosis patients. Cell Stem Cell 2013;13(6):653–8.
21. Wu y, Zhou H, Fan X, et al. Correction of a genetic disease by CRISPR-Cas9-mediated gene editing in mouse spermatogonial stem cells. Cell Res 2015;(25):67–79.
22. Yuan Y, Zhou Q, Wan H, et al. Generation of fertile offspring from Kitw/Kitwv mice through differentiation of gene corrected nuclear transfer embryonic stem cells. Cell Res 2015;25(7):851–63.
23. Milardi D, Grande G, Vincenzoni F, et al. Proteomic approach in the identification of fertility pattern in seminal plasma of fertile men. Fertil Steril 2012; 97(1):67–73.e1.
24. Barceló M, Mata A, Bassas L, et al. Exosomal micro-RNAs in seminal plasma are markers of the origin of azoospermia and can predict the presence of sperm in testicular tissue. Hum Reprod 2018;33(6): 1087–98.
25. Vojtech L, Woo S, Hughes S, et al. Exosomes in human semen carry a distinctive repertoire of small non-coding RNAs with potential regulatory functions. Nucleic Acids Res 2014;42(11):7290–304.
26. Sharma R, Agarwal A, Mohanty G, et al. Proteomic analysis of seminal fluid from men exhibiting oxidative stress. Reprod Biol Endocrinol 2013;11(1):85.
27. Wang Y-X, Wang P, Feng W, et al. Relationships between seminal plasma metals/metalloids and semen quality, sperm apoptosis and DNA integrity. Environ Pollut 2017;224:224–34.

28. Friemel C, Ammerpoh O, Gutwein J, et al. Array-based DNA methylation profiling in male infertility reveals allele-specific DNA methylation in PIWIL1 and PIWIL2. Fertil Steril 2014;101(4):1097–103.e1.

29. Sarkar S, Sujit KM, Singh V, et al. Array-based DNA methylation profiling reveals peripheral blood differential methylation in male infertility. Fertil Steril 2019; 112(1):61–72.e1.

30. Schütte B, El Hajj N, Kuhtz J, et al. Broad DNA methylation changes of spermatogenesis, inflammation and immune response-related genes in a subgroup of sperm samples for assisted reproduction. Andrology 2013;1(6):822–9.

31. Heyn H, Ferreira HJ, Bassas L, et al. Epigenetic disruption of the PIWI pathway in human spermatogenic disorders. PLoS One 2012;7(10):e47892.

32. Schagdarsurengin U. Developmental origins of male subfertility: role of infection, inflammation, and environmental factors. Semin Immunopathol 2016; 38(6):765–81.

33. Elshal MF, El-Sayed IH, Elsaied MA, et al. Sperm head defects and disturbances in spermatozoal chromatin and DNA integrities in idiopathic infertile subjects: association with cigarette smoking. Clin Biochem 2009; 42(7–8):589–94.

34. Waterland RA, Jirtle RL. Transposable elements: targets for early nutritional effects on epigenetic gene regulation. Mol Cell Biol 2003;23(15): 5293–300.

35. Kitamura A, Miyauchi N, Hamada H, et al. Epigenetic alterations in sperm associated with male infertility. Congenit Anom (Kyoto) 2015;55(3):133–44.

Printed and bound by CPI Group (UK) Ltd, Croydon, CR0 4YY

03/10/2024

01040306-0008